Depression

Eleni Palazidou MD, PHD, MRCP, MRCPSYCH
Consultant Psychiatrist
East London and the City Mental Health NHS Trust
The Royal London Hospital (St Clement's), London, UK

Honorary Senior Lecturer
Queen Mary University and the Institute of Psychiatry, London, UK

Emma Tiffin MBBS, BSc Hons, MRCGP
General Practitioner
Tower Hamlets Primary Care Trust, London, UK

Mosby

MOSBY
An affiliate of Elsevier Science

ISBN 0-7234- 3269-4

First published 2003
Reprinted 2003

Cataloguing in Publication Data
Catalogue records for this book are available from the US Library of Congress and British Library.

Note
Medical knowledge is constantly changing. As new information becomes available, changes in treatment, procedures, equipment and the use of drugs become necessary. The authors and publishers have, as far as it is possible, taken care to ensure that the information given in this text is accurate and up to date. However, readers are strongly advised to confirm that the information, especially with regard to drug usage, complies with latest legislation and standards of practice.

The publisher's policy is to use paper manufactured from sustainable forests

Printed by Grafos S.A. Arte sobre papel, Spain.

Contents

Introduction

Abnormal mood states have been recognized since ancient times. Hippocrates described the states of "melancholia" and "mania", attributing the condition of depression (melancholia) to the black bile, one of the four humours he believed responsible for disease. Both these terms survived the passage of time and are still in use today.

The state of melancholia fascinated medical and lay authors and the connection with suicide was made. Robert Burton, himself a sufferer of depression, wrote about his personal experience and current knowledge on the subject, in his treatise *The Anatomy of Melancholy*, in the earlier years of the 17th century. He is thought to have possibly taken his own life, by hanging, after years of relentlessly recurring episodes of depression.

However, it was not until the 20th century that an authoritative attempt was made at classifying mental disorders. Kraepelin, using the psychopathology and course of illness, coined the term "manic depressive insanity" (mood disorders) and separated this from "dementia praecox" (schizophrenia).

The last couple of decades have seen the emergence of internationally accepted classifications of mental disorders (the latest versions being the International Classification for Diseases [ICD-10] and the American Diagnostic and Statistical Manual of Mental Disorders [DSM-IV]) and the introduction of agreed diagnostic criteria. The availability of operational criteria and the development of standardized rating scales have given a major boost to research into the nature and pathogenesis as well as treatment of mental illness, including depression.

Public perception/stigma

Depression is the most widely known, but probably also the most misunderstood, of psychiatric disorders. There is a misconception amongst the public that depression is no different from the common human state of unhappiness and that this is understandable, particularly in the presence of adversity. It has proved difficult to change this attitude. Efforts such as the "Defeat Depression" campaign (1991–1996), jointly launched by the Royal College of Psychiatrists and the Royal College of General Practitioners in the UK, brought about changes in public attitudes in the magnitude of 5–10%. However, MORI (Market and Opinion Research International) polls conducted before and after the campaign showed no difference in the number of lay people that believed psychosocial problems were responsible for depression (less than half considered depression to be an illness; MORI, 1991 and 1997).

A substantial number of depression sufferers fail to seek professional help, partly for the reasons discussed above and partly for fear of the "stigma" of mental illness. In a multicentre European study (the Depression Research in European Society, or DEPRES, study) only 30% of patients, identified as suffering with major depressive disorder in the preceding 6 months, consulted healthcare professionals.[1]

Recognition

In most countries, the majority of patients with depression present to, and are assessed and managed by, primary-care practitioners. Studies in primary care have shown that up to 50% of patients with depression are not detected,[2,3] and these patients appear to have milder disorders and function better than detected patients.[4,5] Little difference in long-term outcome (more than 12 months) has been shown between detected and undetected patients with depression in primary care,[3,5] suggesting that improvement in recognition alone is not enough to improve long-term outcome for depressed patients, and a joint approach to improve both the recognition and management of depression would be needed.

Recognition of depression is also poor in secondary-care non-psychiatric hospital settings where depression is a common psychiatric diagnosis (12.8%). Only 50% of ICD-10 cases of depression are identified by hospital doctors and only half of these are referred for psychiatric opinion.[6]

Inadequate treatment

Low antidepressant use is associated with high suicide rates. In the Jamtland study in Sweden (a survey of the prescription database and suicides between 1970 and 1984), only one-tenth of patients seen by a doctor in the 3 months prior to suicide had received antidepressants and these were often prescribed in low doses.[7]

Despite the advent of antidepressants with lower toxicity and relative safety in overdose, prescribing remains disappointingly low. In the DEPRES study, 30% of patients seen by healthcare professionals were prescribed antidepressants while 17% were treated with benzodiazepines.[8]

Impact on life

It is well recognized that untreated depression is associated with significant functional impairment, which results in increased disability and reduced quality of life for sufferers and their families. Although there is no real increase in the prevalence of depression,[9] it is estimated that by the year 2020, major depressive disorder will be the second most common cause of disability after heart disease.[10]

From an economic perspective, the costs of depression are enormous. In the UK, the cost of drugs for the treatment of depression is 1.9% of the National Health Service pharmaceutical budget. The estimated direct healthcare costs in England and Wales amount to 420 million pounds per year, while indirect costs, generated mostly through loss of productivity, may exceed 3 billion pounds.[11] In the US, the costs of depression are a staggering 43.7 billion dollars per year.[12]

Depression is a common and treatable condition, and investing resources in improving its recognition and management is likely to improve outcome from both the individual and socio-economic perspective.

Definition, Epidemiology and Course

Definition

Unipolar mood disorder presents with recurrent episodes of depression. In bipolar disorder, depressive states alternate with manic states in an irregular fashion, and some episodes may present with symptoms of both mania and depression (mixed affective state). In both unipolar and bipolar mood disorder, episodes of illness are separated by periods of normal functioning.

The ICD-10 and DSM-IV classifications encourage uniformity in the diagnosis of these conditions worldwide, and facilitate research into their epidemiology, pathogenesis and management. There are very few differences in the terms and diagnostic criteria for depressive states as used by these two classifications (see Table 1).

Prevalence

Numerous epidemiological studies worldwide have estimated the lifetime risk, incidence and prevalence of depression.

- The incidence rate is 1.56% (females 1.98 %, males 1.1%).[13]
- Three large studies have recently estimated the prevalence of depression:
  - The National Comorbidity Survey (a large-scale study involving over 8000 people aged 15–54 in the USA[14]) estimated the lifetime prevalence of major depressive disorder as 17.1% (females 21.3%, males 12.7%).
  - The DEPRES study[1] estimated the 6-month prevalence of major depressive disorder as 6.9% (females 8.7%, males 5.0%).
  - The British Psychiatric Morbidity Survey[15] collected data on prevalence, risk factors and associated disability in household, institutional and homeless samples using standardized assessment techniques. Results showed that

2.1% (2.5% females, 1.7% males; aged 16–64) of people studied had a depressive episode in the past week and 7.7% (9.4% females, 5.4% males) had mixed anxiety/depression.

Depression is the most common psychiatric condition. Unipolar depression is more common in women than in men.

The classification of mood disorders	
ICD-10	**DSM-IV**
Manic episode	*Manic episode*
Depressive episode Mild Moderate Severe without psychotic symptoms Severe with psychotic symptoms	*Major depressive episode*
Bipolar affective disorder Currently manic Currently depressed Currently mixed In remission	*Bipolar disorders* Manic episode Depressive episode Mixed episode
Recurrent depressive disorders Mild Moderate Severe without psychotic symptoms Severe with psychotic symptoms	*Depressive disorders* Single episode Recurrent
Persistent mood states Cyclothymia Dysthymia	Cyclothymia Dysthymia
Other mood disorders Recurrent brief disorder	*Depressive disorders not otherwise specified* Recurrent brief depression

Table 1. The classification of mood disorders.

Suicide rates

It is recognized that completed suicide rates are higher in men compared to women, while the opposite holds for attempted suicide. However, in more recent years a trend towards an increase in suicide attempts in males (47% increase in the 1980s compared to the 1970s) has been noted, while in females there is a 9% reduction, bringing the female to male ratio down from 2.3 to 1.4. Deliberate self-poisoning rates have increased in the late 1980s and early 1990s for both genders, with the greatest rise in women aged 15–24 and men aged 15–39.[16]

Course and outcome

(see review by Angst[17])

Factors influencing course

It is now recognized that although patients generally recover from an individual episode of depression, the long-term outcome is not so good because the illness has the tendency to recur (Table 2), with about 75% of people experiencing further episodes.[18] About 10–20% of depressed patients commit suicide and in 15–20% of cases the condition becomes chronic. A 20-year follow-up study found that after the onset of the illness, 20% of a patient's lifetime was spent in a depressed state, and between episodes many patients suffered residual symptoms of depression.[17]

With each new episode the risk of recurrence increases irrespective of age, gender or type of disorder,[19] and a first episode occurring at a young age (below the age of 20) increases the risk of depression in later life.

Depression is a long-term recurring condition.

Factors influencing outcome (Table 3)

Half of patients suffering with major depressive disorder have a coexisting physical or psychiatric disorder, which adversely affects the outcome of depression. There is particularly high co-morbidity with anxiety disorders, most commonly with panic disorder.[20]

Family history of mental illness in first-degree relatives and low intelligence are associated with poorer long-term outcome in depression.[21] Early-childhood events, social supports and other psychosocial factors may also affect long-term outcome, to a lesser extent.

Particular character traits have been associated with a poorer outcome for depression, and these include high neuroticism, hysterical personality, obsessional traits and social deviation.

Risk of recurrence of depression
75% of depressed patients will suffer more than one episode of illness
20% of their lifetime will be spent in depressed state and they may have residual symptoms in between
The risk of recurrence is higher if they experience the first episode below age 20
With each new episode of depression the risk of recurrence increases
10–20% will commit suicide

Table 2. Risk of recurrence of depression.

Factors influencing outcome of depression
Co-morbidity • physical disease • psychiatric disorder (particularly anxiety)
Family history of mental illness
Psychosocial factors
Low intelligence
Premorbid personality

Table 3. Factors influencing outcome of depression.

Aetiology

Depression is probably the best example of a psychobiological condition brought into existence through a complex interaction of nature and nurture. A wide range of aetiological factors are implicated which include heritability, personality, childhood environment, life events, physical and psychological status, brain biochemistry and hormones. No single physical or psychological factor has been demonstrated to bring about depressive illness by itself. It is reasonable to consider depression as a multifactorial condition, the product of a combination of (a) *constitutional factors* that include genetic factors, perinatal and early life experiences determining a vulnerability to this illness via biochemical and psychological processes, and (b) *stressful events*, probably acting as triggers.

Genetic factors

Twin studies, family and adoption studies confirm the importance of genetic vulnerability in the pathogenesis of depression. However, attempts to identify a single gene for either unipolar or bipolar affective disorder have so far been unsuccessful.

It has been easier to study the genetics of bipolar disorder, which has a fairly uniform clinical presentation and course, compared with unipolar disorder. The risk for the identical twin of an affected proband to develop bipolar mood disorder is 65–70%, indicating a strong genetic contribution but also a role for environmental factors. The wide spectrum of the clinical presentation and severity of unipolar depression has made it more difficult to study and genetic research has concentrated largely on the more severe forms of illness.

The suggestion that depression is heterogeneous with distinct genetic and environmentally determined forms is disputed. It has not been possible to subdivide depression into "genetic" and "non-genetic" or indeed into "pure" or co-morbid (for example with alcohol misuse) forms.[22]

It is more likely that, in keeping with Falconer's[23] "multifactorial polygenic model", a pool of genes contributes additively and acts together with environmental factors in bringing about depression. These factors determine a "liability" to illness with multiple thresholds. The more severe the illness in relatives and the larger the number of family members involved (who share genes and environment), the higher is the individual's risk for developing depression. The estimated risk for depression in first-degree relatives of depression sufferers is 10–15%.

Psychosocial factors

A. Life events

- Research in the late 1960s and 1970s[24–28] confirmed the association of life events with depression.
- The life event may act as a precipitating factor, predisposing factor or may influence the form and severity of depression but play no direct aetiological role.
- Examples of life events associated with depression:
  - Childbirth
  - Marriage
  - Retirement
  - Moving house
  - Bereavement

B. Vulnerability factors

1. Lack of social support.
   - Studies have shown that lack of social support is associated with depression,[29,30] while a recent review highlighted individual variation in the protective effects of social ties on mental health.[31]
2. Low social status.[32]
3. Family history of depression.[33]
4. Family conflict.[34]
5. Childhood adversity,[35] including violence.

Psychological hypotheses

"Learned helplessness" is an animal model of depression which is used to test the efficacy of new antidepressants and has been considered analogous to human depression.

The cognitive hypothesis proposes the presence of a cognitive triad consisting of negative "schemata" or evaluations (of one's self, environment and future) acquired as a result of experience that can be activated by stress and bring about a depressed state.

Physical illness (Table 4)

Certain conditions are more likely than others to bring about depressive symptoms. These include some *viral infections*, for example, viral hepatitis, influenza, glandular fever and HIV.

Endocrine disorders are more closely associated with depressive disorder. Over 50% of people with Cushing's syndrome develop depression. Hypothyroidism is also associated with unipolar depression as well as bipolar disorder.

Neurological disorders, particularly those involving the basal ganglia (Parkinson's disease, Huntington's chorea, stroke, multiple sclerosis or Alzheimer's disease) can also cause depression.

Childbirth

About 50% of women experience the "maternal blues" in the first week after childbirth. This is a benign, short-lived and self-limited state of emotionality and tearfulness, and it resolves within 2–3 days. It should not be confused with the pathological state of *postnatal depression*, which affects 10–15% of women and usually occurs 2–4 weeks after childbirth. The risk of postnatal depression is increased to 24% if there is previous history of depression and is as high as 35% if depression started during the pregnancy. A previous episode of postnatal depression raises the risk for recurrence after subsequent pregnancies to 50%.[36]

Physical disorders associated with depressive illness
Endocrine
Cushing's syndrome
Hypothyroidism
Diabetes mellitus
Hyperthyroidism
Hyperparathyroidism
Neurological disorders
Multiple sclerosis
Parkinson's disease
Huntington's disease
Cerebrovascular disease
Alzheimer's disease
Viral infections
Viral hepatitis
Infectious mononucleosis
Influenza
HIV
Autoimmune disorders
Systemic lupus erythematosus

Table 4. Physical disorders associated with depressive illness.

Biochemical

The advent of the first effective antidepressant drugs and understanding their mechanisms of action has paved the way to the development of biochemical theories attempting to explain the genesis of depression. The observation that drugs such as reserpine and tetrabenazine, which are monoamine-depleting agents, are associated with depressive states and that antidepressants drugs (the tricyclic antidepressants [TCAs] and the monoamine oxidase inhibitors [MAOIs]) increase the concentrations of these amines at the synaptic level led to the development of the "catecholamine hypothesis",[37] followed shortly after by the "indoleamine hypothesis of depression"[38] and the amalgamation of the two, the "monoamine hypothesis of depression". This posits that depression is caused by a reduction in brain concentrations of the monoamines noradrenaline (NA) and serotonin (5-HT). Research evidence provided further support for the basic premise of this theory showing impaired function (decreased activity) of the serotonergic and/or noradrenergic central neurotransmitter systems in depression. All currently available antidepressant drugs act by increasing the activity of one or both these systems.

The nuclei of both the noradrenergic and serotonergic neurotransmitter neuronal systems are located in the brain stem, from where they project widely into the brain and in particular to areas considered to be of importance in mood states. The two main noradrenergic pathways extend from the area of the locus coeruleus in the pons to the thalamus, hypothalamus, the limbic system, subcortical limbic structures, the hippocampus and neocortex (see Figure 1). The serotonergic neuronal cell bodies are located in the midline raphe nuclei and from there they extend via a diffuse network into the basal ganglia, the hypothalamus, limbic forebrain and the cerebral cortex (see Figure 2). The 5-HT neurons are active in a "tonic" fashion with slow constant firing and, together with the noradrenergic projections, are thought to have a modulatory function on the activity of other systems located in the areas they project to and in particular those related to mood states. These two systems interact with each other as well as other brain neurotransmitter systems and this is of relevance to depression and its treatment.

Neuroimaging studies have contributed significantly in improving our understanding of the anatomical and physiological function of the brain in relation to mood, and positron emission tomography (PET) studies showed hypometabolism in the left anterolateral prefrontal cortex in patients with unipolar and bipolar depression.[39]

Hypothalamo-pituitary axis (HPA)

The HPA, the stress axis in man, responds to physical or psychological stress by setting in motion a series of "adaptational responses" in order to maintain homeostasis. As this system is shown to be dysregulated in depression (plasma cortisol concentration is increased and this is not suppressed by dexamethasone), Nemeroff[40] proposed the hypothesis that depression is due to "overactivity of the HPA/stress system".

It is tempting to link these changes to the psychosocial theories of depression and the role of life events. However, it is not yet clear whether the HPA abnormalities are secondary to the state of depression or are aetiologically important.

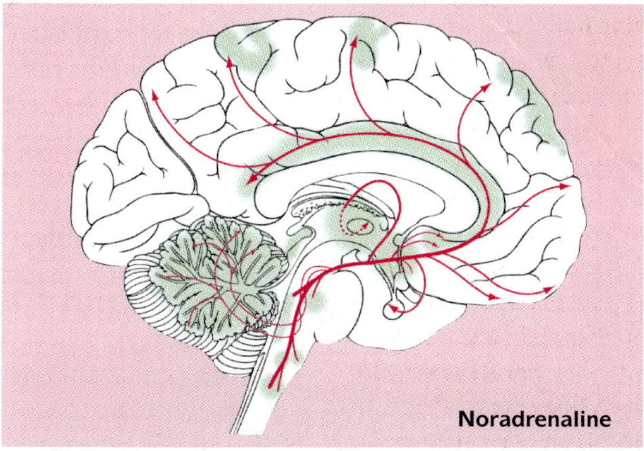

Figure 1. Noradrenergic pathways. Adapted from Carlsson A, Gottfries C-G, Davison A. Neurotransmitters of the brain and ageing. Produced in association with Novartis.

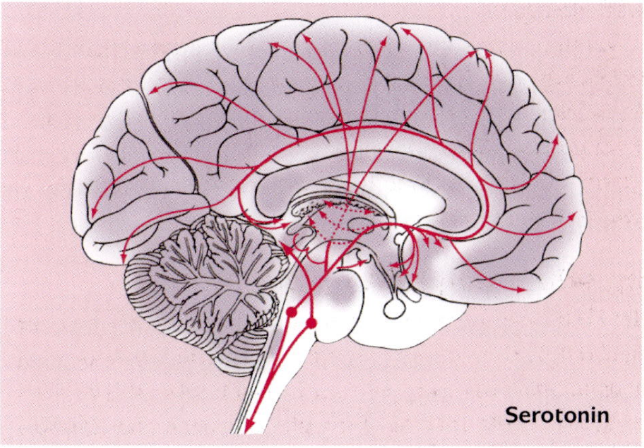

Figure 2. Serotonergic pathways. Adapted from Carlsson A, Gottfries C-G, Davison A. Neurotransmitters of the brain and ageing. Produced in association with Novartis.

Diagnosis

Depression has been subdivided, on the basis of the clinical picture (psychotic or neurotic), the perceived aetiology (endogenous or reactive), severity of illness and other parameters, into subtypes. Most of these subdivisions are rather rigid, unclear and more likely to cause confusion and misconceptions than be of any help in clinical practice, and they are best avoided. However, some subtypes such as atypical depression, psychotic depression, seasonal affective disorder (SAD) and dysthymia are of practical importance mainly because of their preferential response to some treatments, and these will be covered briefly later on in this section.

Making a diagnosis

The diagnosis of depression is based on the criteria required by the ICD-10 and DSM-IV classifications of mental disorders, that are simplified in Table 5 for use in primary care.

Examining the above symptoms/signs in practice may not be as straightforward as it appears. Mood state is a complex state which includes not only subjective feelings of either low or elated mood, but also changes in "cognitions" as well as physiological changes. This abnormal mood state is very different from the normal experience of sadness or elation related to environmental factors (adversity or good fortune). A good understanding of the clinical picture of depression will help the examiner establish the presence/absence of a pathological low mood state and distinguish this from the common and normal human condition of "existential unhappiness".

A thorough assessment of the components of the depressed mood state helps build a clear picture of the patient's condition and a confident diagnosis.

Depressed mood state is very distinct from the normal human state of unhappiness.

Criteria for diagnosis of depression
The presence of the following symptoms, for at least 2 weeks, present most of the time. 1. One or both of the core criteria: • Low or sad mood and/or loss of interest or pleasure (anhedonia) and 2. Some of the following: • Disturbed sleep • Guilt or worthlessness or pessimism • Fatigue or low energy • Disturbed appetite or weight change (more than 5% in 1 month) • Poor concentration or indecisiveness • Psychomotor retardation or agitation • Recurrent thoughts of death or suicidal ideation or attempts

Table 5. Criteria for diagnosis of depression.

Mood as a subjective feeling

Quality

In the "classical" form of depressed state, the subjective feeling of low mood is typically distinct from "normal sadness"; many but not all patients experience it or describe it as such. In practice, patients' description of their mood depends not only on how they feel, but also on their cultural background, education and command of language. They may describe it as sad, low, unhappy, miserable, feeling empty, etc. Sometimes, patients conceal the mood change from others, maintaining a smiling façade ("masked depression"). In such cases, more reliance is placed on the rest of the clinical picture.

Pervasiveness

In depressed states the mood is "pervasive" – present most of the time and cannot be shaken off.

Diurnal variation

Often, depressed mood shows noticeable changes during the day. Typically, patients feel worse in the mornings and better in the evenings. Sometimes, the opposite may be noted.

Reactivity

This is a very useful criterion in distinguishing abnormal mood from unhappiness. Reactivity of mood is impaired in depressed patients – they are not able to react appropriately to enjoyable events/situations. Depending on the severity of the illness, reactivity of mood may be completely lost.

Anhedonia

Anhedonia means inability to derive pleasure. The patient is unable to get any enjoyment from activities and hobbies, which he/she would normally enjoy. A depressed patient loses zest for living and tends to withdraw from social contact.

The pervasiveness of low mood, impaired reactivity and anhedonia are very useful for distinguishing the pathological depressed state from existential unhappiness.

Depressive cognitions

Depressed patients tend to have negative evaluations of:

- themselves (their perceived ability, appearance, etc.);
- their environment;
- the future.

They see themselves as failures and believe that other people see them in the same light. They feel worthless and lose their confidence. They become pessimistic about the future, expecting the worst most of the time. They foresee failure and misfortune and inevitable deterioration in their health. Their hopelessness is often accompanied by thoughts of death and may progress into suicidal thoughts, plans and attempts.

Physiological changes

Sleep

Typically, the patients suffer with middle insomnia (wake up during the night once or more times and have difficulty going back to sleep) and/or early morning wakening (wake up an hour or earlier than their normal time and are unable to go back to sleep).

Sometimes, patients experience difficulty falling asleep (early insomnia) and feel lethargic during the day.

Appetite

Appetite is typically decreased and patients may lose weight. Sometimes, although appetite is still decreased, patients tend to eat for comfort and may gain weight.

Libido

Interest in sex is reduced and there may be problems with sexual function.

Somatic symptoms

Patients are *lacking in energy* and *feel tired*. They find it difficult to carry out their day-to-day activities and neglect their appearance.

There may be complaints of headaches or other aches or pains, constipation or preoccupation with a particular part of their body. Pre-existing physical disorders may be perceived as more troublesome. The patients may have hypochondriacal ideas, believing that certain parts of their body are not functioning properly or that they have cancer or some other serious disease.

Depressive pseudodementia

Depressed patients often suffer with *poor concentration*, which affects their ability to retain new information. As a result they become "forgetful" and fear that their memory is deteriorating.

Psychotic symptoms

In some cases depressed patients experience psychotic symptoms, usually in the form of *delusions*. The content of these delusions is *congruent with their low mood state*. The most common delusions are of guilt, worthlessness, ill health and poverty. Sometimes, they may experience paranoid persecutory delusions.

Depressed patients can also have hallucinations, usually in the form of "*pseudohallucinations*". They usually take the form of auditory hallucinations which the patients believe are inside their head and they recognize as their own thoughts. Often, they hear the voice of a dead person they were close to (parent, spouse or child) usually calling their name. Characteristically, the content of the hallucinations is mood-congruent. The patients may hear voices telling them they are evil or guilty of something and be urged to take their life.

Agitation

Agitation is prominent in some depressed patients and this is most common amongst older patients. They experience constant worry and repeatedly seek reassurance.

Psychomotor retardation

The patient is physically and mentally slowed down. They vacillate over decisions even about simple or minor issues.

Symptoms from other psychiatric disorders

Anxiety

Depressive patients often experience symptoms of generalized anxiety, panic attacks or agoraphobia.

Obsessive–compulsive disorder (OCD)

Symptoms of OCD can also appear during depressed states, or pre-existing OCD may worsen in association with depression.

Depressive subtypes

Depressive disorder with psychotic symptoms

Patients with this condition may have delusions or hallucinations, the content of which is in keeping with their mood. Such patients require antipsychotic as well as antidepressant treatment and they may be candidates for electroconvulsive therapy; it is advisable they are referred to specialist care.

Atypical depression

This depressive subtype has received different definitions in the USA and Europe. According to the DSM-IV, it is a state of depression with preserved reactivity of mood (person brightens up in response to positive events) associated with hypersomnia, increased eating and weight gain, "leaden paralysis" (heaviness in limbs) and a long-standing pattern of extreme sensitivity to perceived interpersonal rejection that results in significant social or occupational impairment.

Seasonal affective disorder (SAD)

Depression in the context of SAD has a regular and temporal relationship with a particular time of the year (starts in autumn/winter) and remits fully in spring, when it may be succeeded by a manic state. This pattern has to be present in the last 2 years. The presentation of winter depression is atypical in that it is characteristically associated with lethargy and overeating with weight gain.

Although it does respond to antidepressants, the treatment of choice is phototherapy.

Dysthymia

This is a chronic depressive state of at least 2 years duration, which does not meet the full criteria for depression and is not the consequence of a partly resolved depressive illness. Early-onset dysthymia (before age 21) is more likely to develop into a major depressive episode in the future. Dysthymia responds to antidepressant treatment,[41] but so far there is little evidence on the efficacy of psychological therapies.

Mixed anxiety–depression

This is commonly encountered in primary-care settings. It presents with a mixture of depressive and anxiety symptoms, which cause significant distress or impairment but do not meet threshold criteria for either depressive or anxiety disorder.

Assessing severity (Table 6)

Making a clear distinction between mild, moderate and severe forms of depression is often very difficult to do in practice, because this condition follows a continuum from a mild illness to a severe illness. As a result, the boundaries between the triage categories are not clearly demarcated and the categories overlap, as illustrated in Figure 3. Despite the difficulty, professionals are encouraged to triage because evidence-based management decisions are guided by the severity of illness. For example, the evidence shows that patients with mild depression may be treated equally effectively by psychological therapy or antidepressant drug treatment, whereas first-line treatment for patients with severe depression is antidepressant drugs.

Assessing suicide risk

Depression is a potentially lethal condition and despite modern management, 10–15% of depressed people commit suicide. Examining the risk of suicide in each patient should be an essential part not only of the initial clinical assessment, but also of any subsequent meetings with the patient until full symptom control has been achieved (see Figure 4, Table 7).

- *Always ask about suicidal thoughts and plans*
- *There is no evidence that asking about suicide increases risk!*
- *Assess risk factors*

Assessing the severity of depression

Triage of depressive illness into mild, moderate and severe guides decisions on management

The *number* of symptoms, the *severity* of individual symptoms and resulting *disability* are all important when deciding on the severity of depression

Table 6. Assessing the severity of depression.

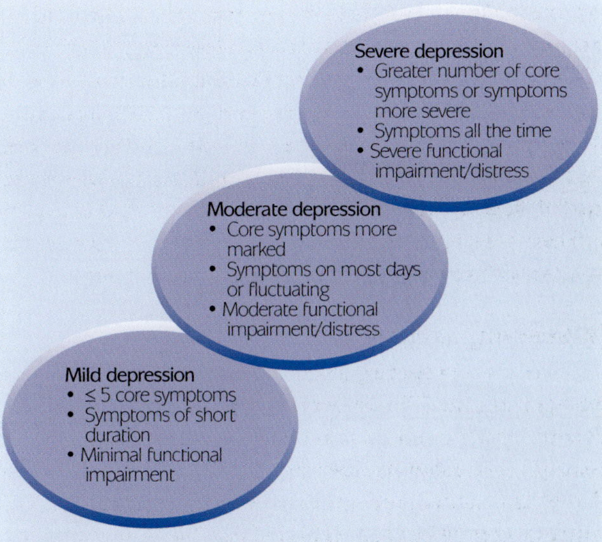

The triage groups are not rigid, and patients may shift between groups during the course of their illness

Functional impairment is defined as being unable to fulfil any one of the following (Kendrick et al., 1994):

- holding down a job
- maintaining self-care and personal hygiene
- performing necessary domestic chores
- participating in recreational activities

Figure 3. Triage categories for depressive illness (symptoms present for *at least* 2 weeks).

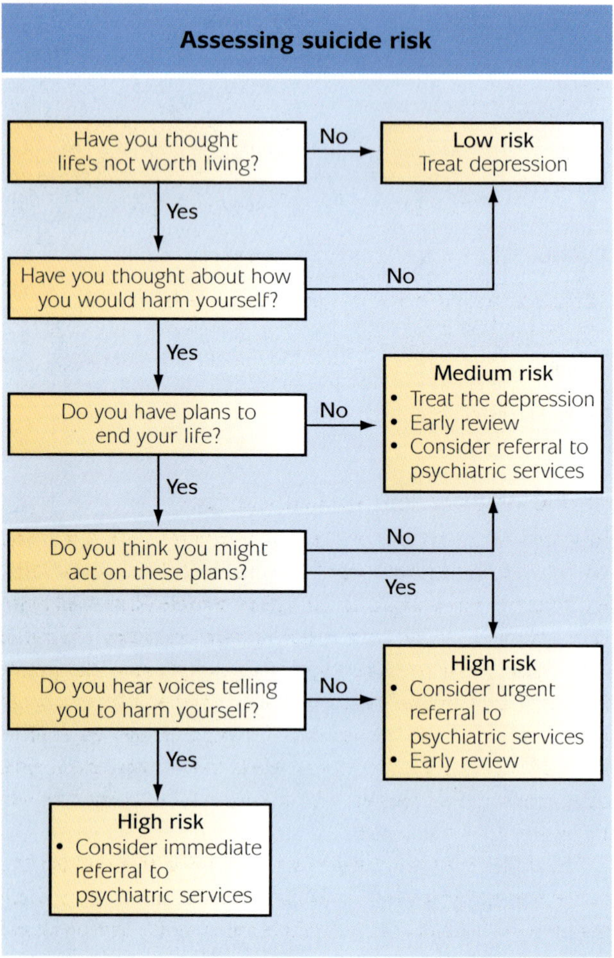

Figure 4. Assessing suicide risk.

Risk factors for suicide	
Demographic Older age Male	*Social* Social isolation Unemployment
Clinical Previous suicidal attempt/ self-harm Serious intent Hopelessness/wish to die Depressed mood state Anxiety symptoms History of depressive disorder Family history	*Co-morbidity* Substance misuse Physical illness Psychiatric disorder (i.e. anxiety disorder, schizophrenia) *Other* Access to weapons, drugs, etc.

Table 7. Risk factors for suicide.

Difficulties with identification

Research suggests that the majority of patients with depression do not seek professional help[1,43] and many of those who do find it difficult to talk about their condition. Patients may feel more comfortable to focus on physical symptoms, partly because they consider them more legitimate complaints, and partly because they fear that professionals may not pay them enough attention if they talk about their feelings. However, studies have shown that patients are more likely to have a psychological assessment if they present with psychological symptoms and for psychological reasons.[44]

There is some evidence that strategies to increase the awareness and knowledge of both the public and doctors about depressive disorders and to train doctors in the detection and treatment of depressive disorders are effective,[45–47] providing that the education and training are ongoing. Younger GPs who have an interest or previous experience in mental health and are under less pressure in terms of clinical workload are better at recognizing the presence of mental disorders.[44]

Depression can be difficult to recognize because it may not present with the classical symptoms of depressive illness and the symptoms may be mild.

Practical tips

Presentation of depression

It is important to be aware that depression may present in ways which make it difficult to recognize. For example, the possibility of depression should be considered in patients presenting with the following:

- Widespread pain or pain out of proportion to the physical cause.
- Feeling tired all the time.
- Frequent attendance, often with minor complaints.
- Other psychiatric conditions, e.g. anxiety, drug and alcohol dependency.
- Physical symptoms not explained by disease (somatization).
- Self-neglect (this is often brought to the GP's attention by a third party).

Patient factors associated with low detection rates for depression

Awareness of these factors may prompt extra vigilance in the professional in their assessment. The following have been associated with low detection rates:

- Male sex
- Older age
- Unemployment
- Coexisting physical illness
- Ethnic minority groups

Depression in the elderly

Making a diagnosis of depressive illness in older people is often difficult because thoughts of death, fatigue, loss of libido, sleep disturbance and pains may all occur more frequently even in the absence of depression. There is also evidence that the common symptoms of depression are less common in older depressed patients (e.g. irritability, loss of interest and finding daily tasks an effort),[48] and communication difficulties and dementing illnesses may add to the problems of identifying those in need of treatment. It is useful to remember that presentations commonly focus on somatic complaints and cognitive deficits.

Depression in patients with coexisting physical illness

Depression may be masked by physical illness. The focus of GP consultations for patients with physical illnesses is often on the illness itself, meaning that there is little time available to address any psychological problems which may coexist or are a consequence of the disease. Studies have shown that patients with cardiovascular or cerebrovascular disease have a higher risk for depression when compared to the general population,[49] and primary-care professionals are well placed to monitor these groups of patients for depression within their chronic-disease management programmes.

Depression in ethnic minority groups

Cross-national epidemiological research has confirmed that major depression occurs worldwide;[50] however, studies based in general practice in the UK have shown that some ethnic minority groups (e.g. Asians) have low consultation rates for depression when compared to the white population.[51] Debate continues on whether the apparently lower rates of depression are due to a genuine difference in prevalence or failure to recognize the illness. There are a number of possible explanations for why it may be difficult to identify depression in the ethnic minorities:

- Presentations may be masked by differences in symptomatic experiences, which are not well captured by western psychiatric concepts and instruments.
- Somatization – there is no conclusive evidence that people from ethnic minority groups are more likely to somatize than the white population and more research needs to be done in this area. The concept that some ethnic minority groups (e.g. Asians and Africans) are more likely to somatize has been based largely on anecdotal observations or research that compares people in different healthcare systems.[52] Some

studies[53–55] have suggested that somatization of depression is ubiquitous, although a recent practice-based study found that Asian patients with depression presented more frequently than white patients with somatic symptoms.[56]

- Stigma – there is evidence of a community stigma associated with mental illness and there is some evidence that women from non-white groups have a fear of being misunderstood by health professionals, leading to a preference for private coping strategies.[57]
- There are no direct equivalents in many languages (e.g. Bengali and Somali) for the term “depression”. This may lead to an incongruity between the term “depression” and its relevance for patients and health workers.

Management

There are three important areas to consider in the management of depression:

- Consultation process and content
- Psychological therapies
- Pharmacological therapies

Consultation process and content

- How the doctor conducts the consultation is an essential part of the management of depression.
- Supportive doctor care alone may be sufficient to resolve mild depressive symptoms, which do not meet the full criteria for depression.
- In patients with mild depressive illness, psychological therapies are as effective as drug treatment in the first 12 months.
- Patients with moderate to severe depressive illness are likely to need drug treatment.

Establishing a therapeutic alliance between the patient and professional

Using consultation skills such as those listed in Table 8 should help to achieve a good working relationship with the patient.

Providing support and advice on the management of depression

Some helpful tips are listed in Table 9.

Explaining depression

Everyone has a different way of explaining depression to the patient, but it is important to avoid medical jargon and to use words that the patient can understand.

Consultation skills important for the recognition and management of depression
Good eye contact
Open-ended questions
Use some directive psychological questions, e.g. "Have you felt low in mood?", "Have you had difficulty concentrating?"
Unhurried, warm, empathic style
Observe patient's non-verbal behaviour and follow up non-verbal cues, e.g. ask about depression if the patient appears tearful or their affect is flat
Follow up verbal cues, i.e. reflect on and use the patient's answers
Positive consultations
Flexible consultation length (single or double appointment): patients often need longer consultations if they are depressed
Continuity of care

Table 8. Consultation skills important for the recognition and management of depression.

Helpful tips to consider including in the consultation
An explanation for depression
Guidance on current problems
Encouragement to develop social support, e.g. self-help groups*
Advice on structured activity and regular exercise (patients may find that keeping an activity diary provides encouragement to do this)
Advice on relaxation and stress management techniques (available in books, or local classes may teach these techniques)
Encouragement to take up hobbies for enjoyment or to build up confidence
Advice on self-help exercises,* e.g. problem solving, where the patient is encouraged to focus on potential solutions to a problem
Recording achievements and/or successes
Provision of written information, e.g. leaflets and books about depression
*It should be remembered that patients with severe depression are likely to need antidepressant treatment before they feel able to carry out self-help activities.

Table 9. Helpful tips to consider including in the consultation.

Examples of explanations:

"Everyone finds that their mood goes up and down but when a person is depressed they find that they feel low all or most of the time and they may find that they don't feel up to doing the things that they usually do, such as working and enjoying their hobbies."

"Depression is a very common condition. Everyone may feel low at some time in his or her lives in relation to circumstances, but that usually passes. It becomes an illness when you are not able to shake it off, however much you try alone or with the support of friends or family. At this point you need professional help and depending on how ill you are, how long you have been depressed and other factors you may need psychological or drug treatment or both of these. The medication helps correct the imbalance of chemicals in the brain."

It is important that both the patient and the family are aware of, and comfortable with, the following ideas:[58]

- Depression is common, and effective treatments are available.
- Depression is an illness and patients with depression are not idle or weak, but they cannot overcome their symptoms without professional help.
- Stress and worry have many physical and psychological effects.

Psychological therapies (see Table 10)

- Always consider psychological therapy as a treatment option for depression.
- The effectiveness of psychological therapies depends upon a good working relationship between the patient and therapist.
- There is no evidence that gender, age, ethnicity or socio-economic status affect the outcome of psychological therapies.
- Patient preference should inform treatment choice (i.e. medication or talking therapy), particularly where the research evidence does not indicate a clear choice of therapy.

Common psychological therapies

Therapy	For whom?	By whom?	Common length of therapy	Evidence of effectiveness	Other comments
Problem solving	Most evidence for mild to moderate depression	Counsellors, trained members of the primary-healthcare team	2–3 brief sessions	Evidence shows short-term effectiveness	–
Counselling	Most evidence for mild to moderate depression	Trained counsellors	Tailored to patient, but usually 6–12 sessions	Evidence shows short-term effectiveness	Particular benefit in helping patients deal with social problems
Cognitive behavioural therapy (CBT)	Most evidence for mild to moderate depression	Clinical psychologist and other trained professionals	Weekly/fortnightly for a contracted number of sessions, e.g. 8–20	Evidence from trials that CBT is as effective as drug therapy in the short term and may be a useful adjunct in the prevention of relapse	–
Psychodynamic therapy	Any degree of depression with composite problems	Professionals trained in psychotherapy	Months to years	Evidence suggests effectiveness. May be a useful adjunct in the prevention of relapse.	Not offered in the acute situation. May be individual/couple/group work.
Interpersonal therapy	Most evidence for mild to moderate depression	Psychotherapist	10–15 sessions	RCTs* show evidence of effectiveness. May be a useful adjunct in the prevention of relapse.	–

* Randomized controlled trials

Table 10. Common psychological therapies.

Psychological therapy is a term used to describe many models of treatment where the common feature is "talking therapy". The term includes both counselling and psychotherapy.

Types of psychological therapy are:

- Type A (integral): general psychotherapeutic skills provided by any mental-health worker within a multidisciplinary package.
- Type B (generic): a psychological treatment package involving a range of techniques from different treatment models. The therapy is tailored to the individual. Health service therapists often use generic psychological therapy.
- Type C (formal): a clearly delineated psychological treatment package based on the theory of psychological treatments where different treatment interventions are used to achieve goals. Type C therapies range from focused (e.g. cognitive behavioural therapy) to more exploratory (e.g. dynamic or analytical therapies) treatments.

1. Structured problem solving

What is it?

- The rationale is that emotional symptoms are caused by problems in everyday life and if these problems are dealt with effectively the symptoms will improve.
- It involves encouraging the patient to identify specific problems, to rank them in terms of importance, and then to focus on one problem at a time, writing down potential solutions and specific steps that he or she might take to implement the solutions.

Who is it for?

- Patients with all grades of depression, but there is most evidence for patients with mild to moderate depression.

Evidence of effectiveness

- There is evidence that problem-solving therapy is effective in the short term (less than 12 months).[59]

2. Counselling

What is it?

- Counselling has been defined as "a systematic process, which gives individuals an opportunity to explore, discover and clarify ways of living more resourcefully, with a greater sense of well-being. Counselling may be concerned with addressing and resolving specific problems, making decisions, coping with crises, working through conflict, or improving relationships with others."[60]
- In simplistic terms, counselling provides a supportive and non-judgemental atmosphere for people to talk over their problems and in general it deals with specific life situations.

Who is it for?

- There is most evidence for patients with mild to moderate depression, particularly if associated with psychosocial issues (e.g. family problems, bereavement, interpersonal difficulties [assertion, self-confidence, problems of intimacy]).
- It is suitable for patients with recent onset (less than 1 year) of depression who would prefer brief treatment.

Evidence of effectiveness

- A Cochrane Review has shown that counselling is effective in the short term (less than 6 months).[61]

3. Cognitive behavioural therapy (CBT)

What is it?

- CBT is based on the belief that depressed people have developed a negative picture of themselves which is self-sustaining.
- CBT aims to replace negative thinking with a more positive attitude to life, more positive behaviours and hence more

positive feelings. It aims to teach patients skills which they can use in any future episodes.
- It is not necessary to identify specific psychosocial issues.

Who is it for?
- There is most evidence for patients with mild to moderate depression, especially if this is associated with negative thinking about self or others.
- Suitable for patients with a history of depression of at least 6 months duration.

Evidence of effectiveness
- A Cochrane Review has shown that CBT is effective in the short term (less than 12 months).[62]

4. Interpersonal therapy (IPT)

What is it?
- IPT focuses on the connection between the onset of depressive symptoms and *current* interpersonal problems. It concentrates on the patients' social situation and dysfunction rather than their personality.

Who is it for?
- Patients with all types of depression but most evidence for patients with mild to moderate depression.

Evidence of effectiveness
- Shown to be effective in the treatment of depressive illness.[63]

5. Psychoanalytical therapy

What is it?
- A number of different therapies based on psychoanalytical ways of understanding human development (Freud and his successors).
- Focal psychodynamic therapy "identifies a central conflict arising from early experience that is being re-enacted in adult life producing mental health problems. It aims to

resolve this through the vehicle of the relationship with the therapist giving new opportunities for emotional assimilation and insight."[60]

- Psychoanalytical therapy "is a longer process (usually a year or more) of allowing unconscious conflicts opportunity to be re-enacted in the relationship with the therapist and, through interpretation, worked through in a developmental process."[60]

Who is it for?

- People who have long-standing interpersonal difficulties and personality problems. It can help people who are cut off from their feelings, feel stuck in their lives and are repeating self-destructive or self-limiting patterns of behaviour.
- Suitable for any symptomatic presentation where the problem can be understood in terms of the person's life circumstances or way of viewing the world.
- The person must have an interest in self-exploration and adequate capacity to tolerate frustration.[60]
- It is not usually offered in an acute situation.

Evidence of effectiveness

- There is evidence of effectiveness.[64]

Common queries

How do we decide whether to treat a depressed patient with psychological therapy or antidepressants?

Psychological therapies, antidepressants and the combination of the two appear equally effective in patients with mild to moderate depressive illness,[65] and the choice depends on clinical judgement and patient preference. However, there is uncertainty with regard to the relative efficacy of psychological therapies compared to drug treatment in patients with severe depression, and drug treatment is advocated with the option of adding psychological therapy if appropriate once the symptoms of depression start to improve.

Evidence suggests that many patients with depression would prefer psychological therapy to drug treatment,[66] and patient preference should inform treatment choice where the research evidence does not indicate a clear choice of therapy.[60]

Which psychological therapy is the most effective?

Controlled trials have shown the following psychological therapies to be effective in the treatment of depression in the short term (less than 12 months):

- Counselling
- Cognitive behavioural therapy (CBT)
- Problem-solving therapy
- Interpersonal therapy (IPT)

There appear to be few significant differences between the types of psychological therapy,[67] although there is evidence for CBT, and a recent Cochrane Review[62] did find that CBT was more effective than other brief psychotherapies.

Do a patient's age, sex, social class and ethnic group affect how they benefit from psychological therapy?

There is no conclusive evidence that the outcome of psychological therapy is affected by the above factors. Psychological therapies should always be considered as a treatment option.

Should we match patients to therapists from the same ethnic minority group?

Reviews on ethnicity suggest that cultural sensitivity by the therapist is more important than ethnic matching of the therapist and patient.[60]

How long should psychological treatment go on?

This is a difficult question because there has been little research looking at the optimal length of psychological treatment. In practice, it is usually determined by local policy and funding, and the average length of treatment in the NHS is eight to 20 sessions. Chronic problems (e.g. chronic relapsing depression) may require longer-term therapy.

Does maintenance psychological therapy prevent the recurrence of depression?

There is some evidence that maintenance psychological therapy may benefit those with chronic depression.[68]

Is psychological therapy cost-effective?

There are few good-quality studies looking at the cost-effectiveness of psychological therapies and this area has been identified as a priority for further research.[60]

Pharmacological therapies

History

Effective antidepressant drugs have been available since the late 1950s, when the first monoamine oxidase inhibitor (MAOI), iproniazid, and the first tricyclic antidepressant (TCA), imipramine, were developed. These drugs were discovered by chance and are a tribute to the observational powers of the clinicians of the time, who noted antidepressant effects in drugs developed to treat completely different disorders (iproniazid was developed as an antituberculous agent and imipramine as an antipsychotic). Once the pharmacology of these earlier agents was worked out it became possible to develop more such drugs.

Until the late 1980s, these two groups of antidepressants were the mainstay of the pharmacological treatment of depression. However, progress in the understanding of the function of the monoamine neurotransmitter systems in the brain, their distribution and interactions and the biochemical/pharmacological and behavioural importance of their neuroreceptors allowed the development of more sophisticated antidepressant drugs.

The last decade saw a proliferation of antidepressants with more selective action, targeting systems presumed to be important in the treatment of depression. The increased selectivity may not have achieved a dramatic increase in efficacy, in general, but it has improved tolerability, as the newer drugs are associated with less side-effects.

Mechanism of action

Despite the large variety of antidepressant drugs, with differing chemical structures, their site and mode of action are fairly limited. They all act on monoamine systems, influencing primarily serotonergic and adrenergic neurotransmission. They increase the availability of serotonin (5-HT), noradrenaline (NA) or both, at the synaptic level, by means of monoamine oxidase inhibition (MAOIs), re-uptake inhibition (TCAs and SSRIs) or $alpha_2$ receptor blockade (Table 11). These actions occur early in the treatment (within hours) and continue for the duration of therapy. After continued exposure to these actions, a number of adaptive changes take place, consisting of an increase or decrease in the sensitivity (up- or down-regulation) of a variety of receptors within the noradrenergic ($beta_1$ and $alpha_1$ adrenoceptors, and $alpha_2$ autoreceptors) and serotonergic (5-HT_{1A} and 5-HT_2 postsynaptic receptors, 5-HT_{1A} somatodendritic receptors and $alpha_2$ heteroreceptors) neurotransmitter systems. Whether some or all of these later effects are simply adaptive changes of no therapeutic value or have major importance in bringing about improvement of the mood state remains to be shown.

Categories of antidepressants

Based on their acute mode of action, antidepressant drugs can be subdivided into the following three major categories:

Pharmacological actions of antidepressant drugs		
	Acute mechanism of action	**Undesirable pharmacological actions**
TCAs Amitriptyline Imipramine Clomipramine Lofepramine Other	NA and 5-HT re-uptake inhibition	Anticholinergic; antihistaminic; $alpha_1$ adrenoceptor blockade; direct membrane stabilization
SSRIs Citalopram (Cipromil) Fluoxetine (Prozac) Fluvoxamine (Faverin) Paroxetine (Seroxat) Sertraline (Lustral)	5-HT re-uptake inhibition	–
MAOIs Phenelzine (Nardil) Isocarboxazid (Marplan) Tranylcypromine (Parnate)	Inhibition of MAO-A and MAO-B isoenzymes	Interaction with tyramine and sympathomimetic drugs; irreversible and non-selective inhibition of MAO isoenzymes
RIMAs Moclobemide (Manerix)	Reversible inhibition of MAO-A	–
SNRIs Venlafaxine (Efexor)	5-HT and NA re-uptake inhibition	–
Reboxetine (Edronax)	NA re-uptake inhibition	–
Nefazodone (Dutonin)	$5\text{-}HT_2$ receptor blockade and 5-HT re-uptake inhibition	–
Mirtazapine (Zispin)	$Alpha_2$ adrenoceptor blockade $5\text{-}HT_2$ receptor	–

Table 11. Pharmacological actions of antidepressant drugs.

- *Monoamine oxidase inhibitors* (Figure 5)
  - Non-selective, non-reversible monoamine oxidase inhibitors (MAOIs)
  - Selective reversible monoamine oxidase inhibitors (RIMAs)
- *Monoamine re-uptake inhibitors* (Figure 6)
  - Non-selective NA and 5-HT re-uptake inhibitors (TCAs)
  - Selective 5-HT and NA re-uptake inhibitors (SNRIs)
  - Selective 5-HT re-uptake inhibitors (SSRIs)
  - Selective NA re-uptake inhibitors (NARIs)
- *Receptor-selective antagonists* (Figure 7)
  - Alpha$_2$ adrenergic receptor antagonists (mianserin and mirtazapine)
  - 5-HT$_2$ serotonin receptor antagonists (trazodone and nefazodone)

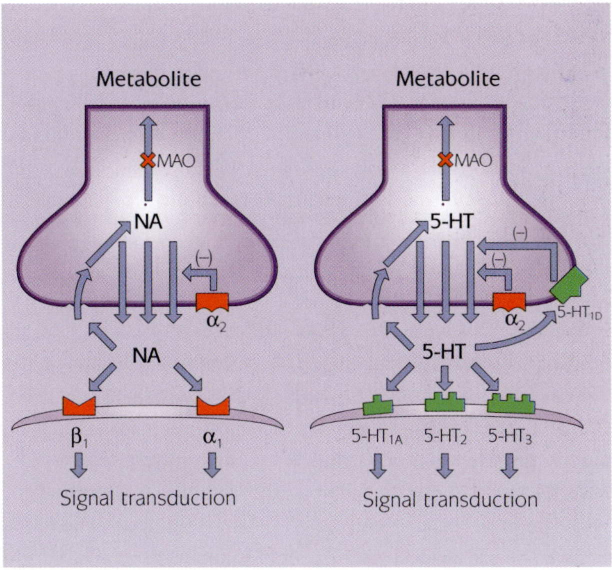

Figure 5. MAOIs and RIMAs inhibit metabolism of NA and 5-HT.

Monoamine oxidase inhibitors

Non-reversible/non-selective monoamine oxidase inhibitors (MAOIs)

Three MAOIs have been available in the UK, the hydrazine derivatives, phenelzine and isocarboxazid, and tranylcypromine, which is amphetamine-like in its chemical structure.

They are useful antidepressants, particularly in the treatment of atypical depression.[69]

Mechanism of action

The target of these drugs is monoamine oxidase (MAO), the enzyme responsible for the intracellular metabolism of 5-HT, NA, dopamine (DA) and some other brain amines. MAO is located within the neuronal terminal, in the outer mitochondrial membrane of storage vesicles. It has an important role to play in regulating the amount of 5-HT and NA available for release by the neuronal terminal in response to neuronal firing. It exists in two isomeric forms, as MAO-A and MAO-B.

The MAOIs exert their effect in blocking the action of this enzyme by irreversibly binding with both isoenzymes. Inactivation of the MAO allows monoamines to accumulate so that larger concentrations can be released, resulting in more powerful stimulation of relevant postsynaptic receptors.

Interactions

MAO blockade has the potential of serious and indeed life-threatening consequences if the subject is exposed to certain agents, which would normally be metabolized by this same enzyme. Prescribing MAOIs therefore requires care, ensuring that patients are given written instructions with advice on dietary requirements and drugs to avoid. For these reasons, the MAOIs are no longer considered as first-choice antidepressants. Nevertheless, there are a relatively small number of patients who were prescribed these agents many years ago and are reluctant to change treatment; therefore, the physician needs to be familiar with these drugs in order to supervise their use safely.

"Cheese reaction"

Tyramine, contained in certain foodstuffs, is normally metabolized by MAO in the gastrointestinal tract. Blockade of this enzyme during treatment with an MAOI allows tyramine to be absorbed, intact, in the general circulation, encouraging release of NA and adrenaline from sympathetic nerve terminals and the adrenal medulla. This increases the concentration of these monoamines (which are already raised due to inactivation of the intraneuronal MAO) and may cause a "hypertensive crisis". The tyramine effect or "cheese reaction" develops within 30 minutes to 1 hour after ingestion of the food, and in its severe form it causes headache, hypertension, palpitations, dilated pupils, motor agitation and other symptoms (Table 12).

Sympathomimetic agents

Similar effects may occur if other sympathomimetic agents, some analgesics, narcotics and TCAs are used concomitantly with the MAOIs (Table 13).

Foodstuffs (high in tyramine) to avoid with MAOIs
Cheese
Meat extracts (Bovril, Oxo)
Broad beans
Marmite
Yeast extracts
Banana skins
Liver
Sauerkraut
Monosodium glutamate
Pickled fish
Red wine
Port
Sausage
Salami

Table 12. Foodstuffs (high in tyramine) to avoid with MAOIs.

Drugs to avoid with MAOIs		
Drug	**Interaction**	**Comment**
Other MAOIs	↑Side-effects, convulsions	Allow 1–2 weeks washout
TCAs	↑Blood pressure, convulsions	Allow 2 weeks washout (may be used in refractory depression with caution)
Carbamazepine (low potential for interaction)	↑Blood pressure, convulsions	Allow 2 weeks washout
SSRIs	Serotonin syndrome	Allow 2 weeks for MAOI washout; 5 weeks for fluoxetine
Amphetamines, methylphenidate	↑Blood pressure	Avoid combination
Some anaesthetics – meperidine	↑Blood pressure, ↑t°, coma	–
Dextromorphan (in Actifed)	Reports of brief psychosis	Avoid high doses
Direct sympathomimetics, e.g. L-dopa	↑Blood pressure	Avoid if possible
Indirect sympathomimetics	Possible hypertensive crisis	Avoid
Hypoglycaemics	May ↑hypoglycaemia	Monitor blood sugar
Fenfluramine, L-tryptophan	Serotonin syndrome	Avoid

Table 13. Drugs to avoid with MAOIs.

Washout period

The irreversibility of the binding of the enzyme is a further problem. Although the concentrations of the MAOIs fall rapidly on discontinuation of treatment, their effects continue until enough new, unbound MAO is synthesized. This takes 2 weeks and it is advisable for the dietary and other restrictions to continue until this time has elapsed. After discontinuing an MAOI, a washout period of at least 2 weeks should be allowed before starting medications likely to interact adversely with the MAOIs.

Side-effects

Some MAOI side-effects become apparent in the early stages of treatment, while others develop during long-term treatment.

- The MAOIs have the potential for *orthostatic hypotension*, although the mechanism for this, unlike the tricyclics, is not related to $alpha_1$ receptor blockade.
- *Weight gain* can be a problem and it occurs in about half of the patients during maintenance treatment with the hydrazine MAOIs (particularly phenelzine), but not with tranylcypromine.
- *Sexual dysfunction* can present in the form of anorgasmia, delayed ejaculation, decreased libido or impotence.
- *Insomnia* is another side-effect appearing later in treatment.
- Although *liver enzymes* are raised in 3–5%, hepatotoxicity is rare.
- *Peripheral neuropathy* is a rare adverse effect caused by pyridoxine deficiency, which can develop during long-term treatment with MAOIs;[70] it is advisable to give these patients pyridoxine.

Indications

The MAOIs are effective antidepressants in depressive illness in general and appear to be more effective than the tricyclics in the treatment of atypical depression.[69] They have also been used in resistant depression, in facial pain and other states.

Reversible monoamine oxidase inhibitors (RIMAs)

Moclobemide (Manerix)

This is the only antidepressant in this group licensed in the UK.

Mechanism of action

It is primarily a MAO-A inhibitor and its binding to the enzyme is reversible.

Interactions

The selective and reversible action of moclobemide means that it has no major interactions with tyramine, although there may be mild clinical manifestations of a "cheese reaction". It is advisable to take moclobemide after food to minimize this risk. Similarly, there are no significant interactions with other drugs apart from narcotics, particularly meperidine.

Side-effects

Its side-effect profile is very good and no toxicity in overdose is seen (up to 20 g). It does not encourage weight gain.

Indications

Moclobemide is effective in all forms of depression. It has also been shown to be effective in the treatment of social phobia.[71]

Monoamine re-uptake inhibitors

Tricyclic antidepressants (TCAs)

This is the largest group of antidepressants, which have a common core chemical structure in the form of a tricyclic ring but different side chains. The latter have a major role in the pharmacological actions of the TCAs and the differences between them.

The deamination of the tertiary amines to the secondary amines is associated with significant changes in their respective potencies on NA and 5-HT re-uptake, as well as direct receptor effects.

Mechanism of action

The common acute pharmacological action of all TCAs, which is responsible for their antidepressant properties, is NA and 5-HT re-uptake inhibition. This increases the availability of these monoamines in the synaptic cleft, which results in increased binding of the relevant postsynaptic receptor sites, achieving higher activity in the stimulated neuron.

In addition to their therapeutic action on the monoamine systems, the TCAs have many other pharmacological effects on neural sites not relevant to depression. These include muscarinic receptor blockade, $alpha_1$ adrenergic receptor blockade and histaminic (H_1) receptor blockade. Each one of these actions is associated with a number of side-effects commonly encountered during treatment with TCAs.

Interactions

A working knowledge of the pharmacokinetics and pharmacodynamics of all antidepressant drugs is important for safe and effective prescribing. This knowledge is even more important in the case of the TCAs because of their cardiotoxicity and lethal potential.

Concomitant administration of TCAs and SSRIs

The TCAs are metabolized in the liver by the hepatic microsomal P450 cytochrome enzyme system. Of particular interest is the cytochrome P450 IID6 isoenzyme, responsible for the hydroxylation of drugs such as the TCAs. Cytochrome P450 IID6 is inhibited by some SSRIs (fluoxetine, paroxetine), and concomitant TCA and SSRI administration is likely to increase TCA concentrations, resulting in possible toxicity.

Concomitant use of TCAs and MAOIs

This has potentially dangerous consequences, although these drugs are sometimes used together in resistant depression and can be safe in experienced hands. Nevertheless, it should be noted that clomipramine, because of its powerful 5-HT re-uptake inhibitory properties, should not be combined with MAOIs.

Alcohol

Chronic alcohol use is not uncommon in patients with depression and may increase the metabolism of the TCAs by inducing hepatic enzymes. This may lead to reduced concentrations and possibly efficacy. The opposite may be a problem in the presence of liver cirrhosis/failure.

The pharmacodynamic interactions of the TCAs with alcohol are also relevant, and significant psychomotor and cognitive adverse effects occur when they are taken together.[72]

Side-effects

The many pharmacological actions of the TCAs outside their re-uptake inhibitory properties are responsible for the rather extensive list of side-effects associated with this group of antidepressants (see Table 14). Some of these side-effects, for example sedation or orthostatic hypotension, are more troublesome with tertiary amines than second-generation TCA treatment. In general, they are fairly well tolerated and a source of nuisance rather than concern in young and physically healthy individuals. However, they may cause serious problems to some vulnerable populations, such as the elderly or physically sick.

The TCAs have a narrow therapeutic index and doses only 10 times the therapeutic dose can be toxic. It is important to be aware that about 5–10% of Caucasians (3% Blacks and 1%

Asians) have low CYP IID6 activity[73] and are therefore at risk of accumulating toxic concentrations of TCAs when receiving doses within the therapeutic range.

Antimuscarinic effects

In the elderly, antimuscarinic actions may result in urinary retention in the presence of prostatic hypertrophy, severe constipation and even paralytic ileus. They may cause or worsen cognitive deficits and aggravate narrow-angle glaucoma.

Cardiovascular effects

- There may be *increase in heart rate*, which is probably related to vagal inhibition and possibly also to adrenergic effects (NA re-uptake inhibition).

Side-effect profile of TCAs
Anticholinergic
Dry mouth
Blurred vision
Urinary hesitancy (urinary retention)
Constipation
Memory impairment
Aggravation of narrow-angle glaucoma
Antihistaminic
Sedation
Weight gain
Alpha$_1$ adrenoceptor antagonism
Orthostatic hypotension
Cardiac effects
Cardiovascular effects
Sinus tachycardia
Arrhythmias
Conduction delay
Sudden death
Other side-effects
Sexual dysfunction
Impaired cognitive and psychomotor skills
Convulsions

Table 14. Side-effect profile of TCAs.

- $Alpha_1$ adrenergic receptor blockade is responsible for *orthostatic hypotension*. This may be present with only mild dizziness in the young, but can cause falls in an elderly person.
- It is important to remember that the TCAs' quinidine-like action of membrane stabilization slows conduction. This has no clinical effects in healthy individuals, but may cause *partial or complete heart block* in patients with pre-existing cardiac disease. Patients with ventricular arrhythmias or ischaemic heart disease are at risk of *sudden death*, even at therapeutic concentrations.[74]
- *Sudden deaths* have been reported during treatment with TCAs, in particular desipramine, in children, although the precise mechanism is unclear.[75]
- Their potential for cardiotoxicity renders these antidepressants unsafe in overdose and their use should be avoided in patients at risk of suicide. Lofepramine is the only TCA that is safe in overdose.

Sedation

Sedation is more pronounced during treatment with the tertiary amine TCAs that have more powerful antihistaminic and $alpha_1$ antagonist properties. This may be a problem for many patients, particularly those who drive or work with machinery, but it may be of benefit to others who have severe insomnia and/or agitation.

Weight gain

This is probably related to the antihistaminic action of the TCAs as well as carbohydrate craving and slowing of metabolism, although the mechanism for these is not clear.

Sexual dysfunction

This is more likely to be related to the serotonergic effects of the TCAs and is less of a problem than during treatment with SSRIs.

Indications

The TCAs are effective in depressive illness of any severity. Indeed, in more severe depressed states they are more effective than the SSRIs.[76] This superiority of efficacy is probably related to their dual action, increasing the activity of both the noradrenergic and serotonergic systems. There is, however, some evidence that men respond better to TCAs than women, who show variable response, and the latter is possibly related to oestrogen concentrations.[77]

Patients with atypical depression also show poorer response to TCAs compared to MAOIs.[69]

When the depressive picture is complicated by psychotic features, TCAs alone are not, in general, effective enough and the addition of an antipsychotic is indicated in such cases. Amoxapine, a TCA with antidopaminergic properties, is considered effective in psychotic depression, although in practice, at least in the UK, this is not commonly used.

TCAs are also successfully used in the treatment of chronic pain and enuresis in children.

Selective 5-HT and NA re-uptake inhibitors (SNRIs)

This is a relatively new group of antidepressants, which like the TCAs increase adrenergic and serotonergic activity by blocking 5-HT and NA re-uptake (Figure 6). However, unlike the TCAs they are highly selective and do not have antimuscarinic, antihistaminic or receptor-specific properties. They are also devoid of cardiotoxic effects. The side-effects associated with the SNRIs are due to their serotonergic and adrenergic effects.

Venlafaxine (Efexor)

This is the only SNRI currently licensed in the UK. It has very good bioavailability and low protein binding capacity, unlike most other psychotropic drugs. In average doses it is primarily a 5-HT re-uptake inhibitor and its adrenergic action becomes significant when higher doses are used; this may be the reason why at higher doses blood pressure may be increased in predisposed individuals. In more severe depressed states it is advisable to use higher doses in order to achieve dual action and hence better efficacy.

Milnacipran

Milnacipran is not licensed in the UK, although it is available elsewhere in Europe (France). It appears to have fairly equipotent 5-HT and NA re-uptake inhibitory properties.

Selective serotonin re-uptake inhibitors (SSRIs)

In the last decade, this group of antidepressants has largely replaced the TCAs as first-line antidepressants, despite the unfavourable cost differences. This popularity is related to their side-effect profile, affording better tolerability compared to the TCAs,[78] and their relative safety in overdose.[79] There are several SSRIs licensed in the UK (see Table 11).

Mechanism of action

Unlike the TCAs, the SSRIs have diverse chemical structures but a common substrate for pharmacological action. They enhance serotonergic activity by selectively blocking 5-HT re-uptake (Figure 6) in serotonergic neurons. They do not have direct receptor effects or clinically significant influence on other neurotransmitter systems.

Interactions

The SSRIs have both pharmacokinetic and pharmacodynamic interactions of clinical significance and the prescribing clinician needs to be aware of these.

Pharmacokinetic interactions

Some of the SSRIs have active metabolites, which should be taken into consideration when using these drugs.

- *Fluoxetine* – Norfluoxetine, a metabolite of fluoxetine, is a powerful 5-HT re-uptake inhibitor in its own right and has a longer half-life. This prolongs the elimination period of this SSRI upon discontinuation. It is therefore advised that drugs which interact adversely with fluoxetine, such as the MAOIs, should not be prescribed for at least 5 weeks after it has been discontinued.[80]

- *Sertraline* – This SSRI also has an active metabolite, desmethylsertraline, which is much weaker as a 5-HT re-uptake inhibitor (10 times) than the parent drug, but has a longer half-life.

The SSRIs have important pharmacokinetic interactions with other pharmacological agents through their effects on the hepatic cytochrome enzyme system. The most significant interaction is related to their ability to inhibit cytochrome P450 IID6 that metabolizes drugs such as the TCAs, some antipsychotic and other agents, resulting in raised concentrations of these drugs.[81] Paroxetine and fluoxetine are the most powerful inhibitors.

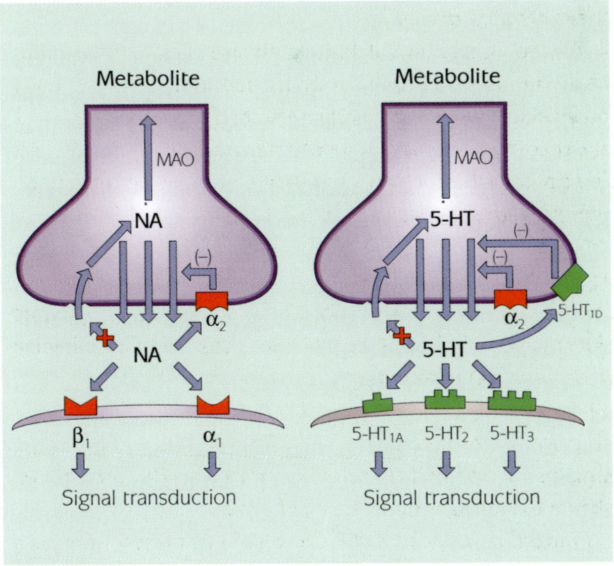

Figure 6. TCAs and SNRIs inhibit re-uptake of both NA and 5-HT. SSRIs inhibit re-uptake of 5-HT.

Pharmacodynamic interactions

The most important of these is their interaction with the MAOIs. The combined action of reuptake inhibition of 5-HT and prevention of its intraneuronal metabolism results in unduly high concentrations of this amine, and serotonergic activity may increase to an unacceptably high level, causing a toxic state, "serotonin syndrome", which can be lethal. Diagnostic criteria are shown in Table 15.[82] Milder forms of this syndrome probably go unrecognized, hence it is assumed to be rare. Excessive activation of serotonergic activity by means of other serotonergic drugs or combinations of such drugs may also cause this syndrome.[83] It is advisable to monitor patients for the early signs of excessive serotonergic activity when SSRIs are used in high doses or in combination with TCAs, in particular clomipramine.

Side-effects

The adverse effects associated with the SSRIs are intrinsic to their serotonergic activity. The increased 5-HT concentrations bind indiscriminately to all 5-HT receptor subtypes available. Stimulation of some of these may not be relevant to the drugs' antidepressant action, but can be responsible for side-effects (see Table 16). For example, nausea, a common side-effect of SSRIs, is due to 5-HT_3 receptor activation, while 5-HT_{1D} activation may be responsible for headache and exacerbation of migraine.

The SSRIs do not have significant effects on non-serotonergic sites, although paroxetine has a small potential for antimuscarinic side-effects.

In general, the SSRIs' side-effects are reasonably well tolerated, which reduces drop-out rates and allows immediate prescribing of an effective therapeutic dose, avoiding the requirement for several days of upward titration as for the TCAs.

Serotonin syndrome – suggested diagnostic criteria
A. Coincident with the addition of or increase in a known serotonergic agent to an established medication regimen, at least three of the following clinical features are present: • mental status changes (confusion, hypomania) • agitation • myoclonus • hyperreflexia • diaphoresis • shivering • tremor • diarrhoea • incoordination • fever B. Other aetiologies (e.g. infectious, metabolic, substance abuse or withdrawal) have been ruled out. C. A neuroleptic had not been started or increased in dosage prior to the onset of the signs and symptoms listed above.

Table 15. Serotonin syndrome – suggested diagnostic criteria. Reprinted with permission from reference 82.

Side-effect profile of SSRIs
Nausea/vomiting
Abdominal pain
Dry mouth
Constipation/diarrhoea
Headache
Asthenia
Dizziness
Insomnia/somnolence
Sweating
Anorexia
Weight loss
Nervousness/agitation
Tremor
Convulsions
Dystonic reactions
Sexual dysfunction (reduced libido, anorgasmia)

Table 16. Side-effect profile of SSRIs.

Indications

SSRIs are effective antidepressants and have been the subject of rigorous and extensive investigation through clinical trials. Like the MAOIs, they also have been found to be particularly effective in "atypical depression", but not as effective as the TCAs in more severe forms of depression.

Serotonergic neurons are widely spread within the brain and they are involved in multiple functions. The SSRIs therefore have been found useful in the treatment of a variety of psychiatric conditions in addition to depression (anxiety disorders, obsessive–compulsive disorder, bulimia nervosa, aggression).

Recent evidence suggests that the efficacy of SSRIs may wane over time[84] and a higher dose may be needed to maintain efficacy.

Selective NA re-uptake inhibitors (NARIs)

Reboxetine (Edronax)

Some of the TCAs, such as desipramine, and the tetracyclic maprotiline are potent and relatively selective NA re-uptake inhibitors. Reboxetine is the only NA re-uptake inhibitor devoid of direct serotonergic activity or receptor effects. It is licensed in some countries, including the UK.

By virtue of its selectivity it has a very low potential for side-effects. Unlike the TCAs, it has no direct cardiac effects.

Receptor-selective antidepressants

Alpha$_2$ adrenergic receptor antagonists

Mianserin

Mianserin found a place in the treatment of depression for many years as an alternative to the tricyclics and MAOIs, particularly because of its safety in patients with cardiac problems.

It has the potential for agranulocytosis and its use has waned in recent years.

Mirtazapine (Zispin)

Mirtazapine is an aza analogue of mianserin and has a complex mode of action (see Figure 7), resulting in the activation of both the serotonergic and noradrenergic neurotransmitter systems.

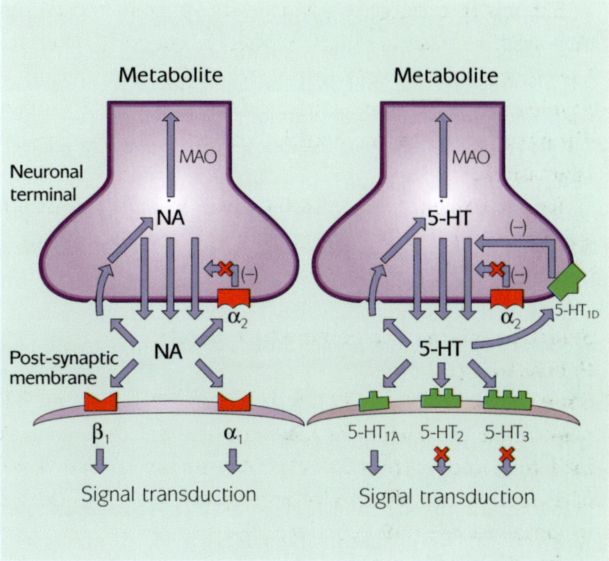

Figure 7. Mirtazapine blocks $alpha_2$ auto- and heteroreceptors on the neuronal terminal and $5\text{-}HT_2$ and $5\text{-}HT_3$ postsynaptic receptors. Trazodone and nefazodone block $5\text{-}HT_2$ postsynaptic receptors.

Mechanism of action

Its primary action involves the blockade of $alpha_2$ autoreceptors on noradrenergic neurons and $alpha_2$ heteroreceptors located on serotenergic neurons, increasing the concentrations of these amines in the synaptic cleft. The blockade of $alpha_2$ somatodendritic adrenergic receptors disinhibits cell firing, increasing the release of NA. The increased noradrenergic activity stimulates further the activity of the serotonergic neurons via $alpha_1$ adrenergic receptors located on the bodies of these cells in the raphe nuclei.

Side-effects

In addition to the above actions, mirtazapine also has direct 5-HT receptor effects, which enhance its antidepressant activity and reduce the potential for some side-effects associated with SSRIs:

- *5-HT_2 receptor blockade* – facilitates transmission of the serotonergic signal via the postsynaptic 5-HT_{1A} receptor, which is thought to be important for antidepressant efficacy. It also reduces the potential for some side-effects such as agitation and sexual problems and improves sleep.
- *5-HT_3 receptor blockade* – reduces the likelihood of nausea.

Mirtazapine also has fairly marked antihistaminic properties, which are probably responsible for sedation and weight gain, common and well-recognized side-effects. These may be a problem for some patients, although for those with significant weight loss and insomnia they may be beneficial. There is some anecdotal evidence that higher doses are associated with less sedation.

5-HT_2 receptor antagonists

Trazodone (Molipaxin)

Trazodone is a mixed agonist/antagonist at 5-HT receptor sites and a weak 5-HT re-uptake inhibitor. It is a modestly efficacious antidepressant, but is useful for its hypnotic and anxiolytic properties.

Its affinity for $alpha_1$ adrenergic receptors may cause orthostatic hypotension and this may be a problem in the elderly. A recognized but rare unpleasant side-effect of this antidepressant is priapism.

Nefazodone (Dutonin)

This is an analogue of trazodone and has a similar mechanism of action.

Mechanism of action

It is a potent 5-HT_2 receptor antagonist and a weak 5-HT re-uptake inhibitor. By blocking 5-HT_2 postsynaptic receptors, like mirtazapine, nefazodone increases transmission of the serotonergic signal via 5-HT_{1A} postsynaptic receptors, hence enhancing the antidepressant effects and reducing the potential for agitation and sexual problems.

Side-effects

It is relatively sedative and well tolerated. Unlike trazodone, it has low affinity for $alpha_1$ receptors and is not associated with priapism.

A flow chart of the drug treatment of depression is shown in Figure 8.

Discontinuation syndrome

Abrupt discontinuation of treatment associated with withdrawal symptoms has been reported with most antidepressants. It is important to remember that withdrawal symptoms are related to all potent pharmacological actions of the drugs concerned and not only those responsible for their antidepressant properties.

For example, on abrupt withdrawal of TCAs, patients can suffer unpleasant symptoms due to increased cholinergic activity ("cholinergic crisis").

Drugs with short half-lives are more likely to cause withdrawal symptoms. These occur in 1–3 days. Paroxetine and venlafaxine have been reported to cause such symptoms, even when patients omit a single dose, while fluoxetine, by virtue of its long half-life and that of its metabolite, is unlikely to have withdrawal effects.

The most common withdrawal symptoms associated with SSRIs are dizziness, nausea, "flu-like symptoms", fatigue, sleep disturbances, anxiety, irritability and crying spells (Table 17).

It should be noted that antidepressant drugs are not associated with dependence and their withdrawal effects, therefore, do not consist of symptoms typical of addictive drugs, for example drug-seeking behaviour.

Antidepressant drugs are not addictive.

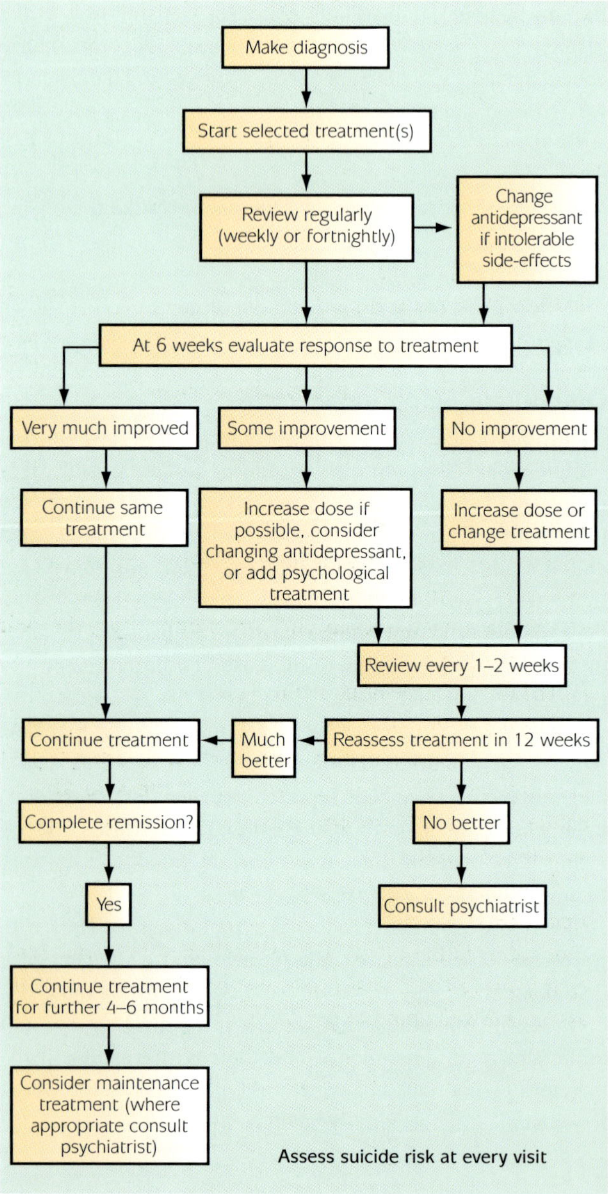

Figure 8. Flow chart – Drug treatment of depression.

Withdrawal symptoms
Withdrawal symptoms might include: Dizziness* Electric shock sensations* Anxiety/agitation* Insomnia Flu-like symptoms Diarrhoea/abdominal spasms Paraesthesia* Mood swings Nausea Low mood *Common in SSRI/venlafaxine withdrawal.

Table 17. Withdrawal symptoms.

Treatment aims

The ultimate aims of treatment should be:

- Complete symptom resolution
- The return to premorbid functioning (psychosocial, occupational)
- The maintenance of normality
- The prevention of recurrence

In order to achieve these objectives, and in keeping with current ideas about the course of depressive illness,[85] antidepressant drug treatment should consist of three phases, as outlined below.

Acute treatment

This refers to the first 6–12 weeks of treatment and aims at *remission* (control of symptoms). Inadequate response is associated with poor prognosis.

Continuation treatment

This is aimed at maintaining remission status and *prevention of relapse*. On the basis of research evidence of high relapse rates during this period, it is recommended that antidepressant drug treatment be continued for 6 months after full symptom control.

The antidepressant drug which achieved remission should be continued in the same dose.

Maintenance treatment

This aims at *prevention of recurrence* of a further episode of depression. Maintenance treatment is indicated in patients who have had previous episodes and are therefore at higher risk of these recurring. The need for maintenance treatment will be influenced not only by the known course of the individual patient's illness, but also by relevant psychosocial factors and the patient's physical health.

There is a misconception that a "maintenance dose" could be safely lower than the "acute treatment dose". Such reduction will expose the patient to an unnecessary risk of relapse.

It is advisable to consult with a psychiatrist when presented with patients likely to need longer-term treatment.

Engaging the patient in treatment

In order to achieve the above aims, it is essential that the patient be involved in a therapeutic alliance. This can be achieved by giving the patient adequate information about the nature of their illness and the need for treatment. A positive message about the treatability of this illness will help engage the patient who, because of the very nature of his/her condition, will often be feeling hopeless about the future. It should be explained that antidepressants are not addictive and that they do not alter one's personality nor affect their intelligence. These are common misconceptions the public have about antidepressant drugs.

Once the patient has agreed to start treatment, the next step is to ensure compliance. If the patient knows that it may take about 2 weeks before his/her symptoms start showing significant improvement, that they may experience some side-effects and they are told what to expect, they will be more likely to adhere to the treatment. A reassurance should be given that the antidepressant could be changed if they are unable to tolerate the original drug prescribed. Regular reviews of the patient's mood state and suicidal risk offers further reassurance and support, helps ensure compliance and allows prompt intervention in the case of any serious worsening of the condition.

Choice of antidepressant

The choice of antidepressant should be tailored to the individual. A good assessment of the patient's mood state and psychosocial conditions, as well as a reasonable knowledge of antidepressants from different groups, will help choose the optimum agent. The following factors should be considered:

- Severity of illness
- Clinical presentation
- Suicidal risk
- Previous response to treatment
- The likely tolerability of potential side-effects
- The likely benefit of potential side-effects, such as sedation
- The likely drawbacks of potential side-effects, such as sedation (i.e. working with machinery, driving, etc.)
- Pregnancy or breastfeeding
- Concomitant treatment of physical illness or other psychiatric disorders with the potential for pharmacokinetic/ pharmacodynamic interactions
- The presence of relevant physical (e.g. cardiovascular) disease

Future Developments

Depression is a recurring, incapacitating, long-term condition. The prediction that, within the next 20 years, it will take second place only to heart disease as the most common cause of disability, is an ominous warning. Its consequences for the sufferers, their families and society and its costs are enormous. Yet this is a treatable disorder. Allocating more resources in the recognition and management of depression will be a wise investment and well worth considering by the fund holders.

Treatments, both pharmacological and psychological, have made major progress in the last decade. Effective psychological therapies which are more focused and short-term have been developed, such as cognitive therapy. The long-term efficacy of such therapies is being examined, with encouraging early results.

Major progress has been achieved in the pharmacological domain. Selective drugs have been developed with better tolerability and safety in overdose. A variety of new drugs are in the process of development, such as SNRIs, RIMAs and receptor-specific agents. Systems other than the monoamines, for example the *N*-methyl-D-aspartate (NMDA) receptor complex, have been implicated in depression and may be the target of effective novel antidepressants. Such approaches may be not only more effective (either alone or in combination with traditional antidepressants), but also achieve a faster onset of action.

Advances in molecular biology and genetics widen the horizons, offering the potential of alternative pharmacological treatment strategies.

Case Histories

Case 1

History

Mr X is a 55-year-old man who complains that he has been feeling down for the last 2 months and he attributes this to stress at work. He works as a heavy-goods-vehicle driver and his hours have been changed to include more night shifts.

He tells you that recently he has not been sleeping well and has been off his food. He also complains of feeling tired all the time, to the extent that he doesn't even feel like going out into the garden (his favourite hobby). He does not have any suicidal ideas. He tells you that his symptoms do not affect his work at present but he is worried that they may do so if there is any deterioration.

Mr X has a wife and two children and he describes the family relationship as good.

Until 2 months ago, Mr X had never had problems with his mood and he has no family history of mood disorder. He drinks 1 pint of beer on weekend nights only and has never experimented with drugs. He is known to have prostatism, but otherwise he is fit and well and not on any other medications.

Discussion

Diagnosis

A diagnosis of major depression can be made because the ICD-10 criteria of depression are fulfilled.

Triage

Currently, Mr X is not disabled by his symptoms and is able to continue working, so a diagnosis of mild depression can be made.

Risk assessment

Mr X has no suicidal ideas but there is a possibility that deterioration in his symptoms could affect his ability to drive. Therefore, regular follow-up is important to monitor depressive symptoms and their effects.

Management options

Social

It appears that this episode of major depression was precipitated by stress at work, and therefore this needs to be addressed and ways of relieving the stress identified, e.g. reducing the number of night shifts worked. It is important to encourage Mr X to discuss his working pattern with his employer and to identify solutions. Mr X may need a short time off work to relieve the immediate pressure and his symptoms may improve spontaneously during this time. His good family relationship is likely to aid his recovery.

Psychological

The focus should be on problem solving (this would involve identifying the problems that Mr X has at work and finding potential solutions) and support. Supportive care by the GP may be sufficient to resolve the symptoms in view of the fact that Mr X has a mild depressive illness. Alternatively, Mr X could be referred to a counsellor or psychologist for short-term therapy (evidence has shown that psychological therapies are only effective within the first 12 months of depressive illness). The diagnosis of depression should be discussed with the patient and reassurance given that the illness is treatable. Providing written information about depression has been shown to aid recovery and this may include suggesting books to read about depression, giving a practice leaflet to the patient, etc.

Drug treatment

The option of antidepressant drug treatment may be discussed with Mr X, but it is likely that his symptoms will resolve with supportive or psychological treatment alone. Discussion about antidepressants should include information on side-effects and duration of treatment. TCAs should be avoided in view of Mr X's history of prostatism and because their side-effects (sedation and blurred vision) may impair driving ability.

Case 2

History

Miss Y is a 42-year-old lady who is complaining that she has been feeling increasingly depressed for the last 3 months. She works in a travel agency and has been taking days off work because she hasn't felt well enough to do her job and she has been avoiding social activities. She says that she no longer enjoys life, she is sleeping badly (she wakes at 3 a.m.) and her appetite is poor. She is unable to relax, finds it difficult to concentrate on work and she keeps feeling guilty about taking time off work. Miss Y also tells you that recently she has felt that she would be better off dead, although she doesn't think that she could ever actually harm herself and has never done so in the past. She lives alone following her divorce 3 years ago and has no close relationships with family or friends.

Miss Y has a history of depression since the age of 16 years and in the last 4 years she has had two episodes of depressive illness. She has been taking amitriptyline (75 mg nocte) for the last 4 years and prior to that she had tried various SSRIs for short periods of time, which she claims did not help her depression. She drinks approximately 20 glasses of wine per week and occasionally smokes cannabis with friends. Her mother had depression. The only medical history of note is episodic palpitations and she takes chlorpromazine occasionally when she feels very anxious.

Discussion

Diagnosis

A diagnosis of major depression can be made because the ICD-10 criteria of depression are fulfilled.

Triage

A diagnosis of moderate to severe depression can be made because Miss Y's symptoms are having a significant adverse effect on her everyday life (she is finding it difficult to work).

Risk assessment

Miss Y has told you that recently she has felt that she would be better off dead, although she doesn't think that she could ever actually harm herself. It is important to assess her degree of hopelessness; the *intrusiveness of suicidal thoughts* and whether she has thought about a *suicide plan*, as these would both increase her risk. It is also important to exclude any *psychotic symptoms*. Obtaining a detailed *drug and alcohol history* is also important. Cannabis can exacerbate depression and Miss Y should be informed of this. Drinking 20 units of alcohol/week is only just over the recommended amount for women (14 units/week), but the pattern of drinking, e.g. if she binges, may increase risk. *Living alone* is another risk factor and Miss Y does not appear to have any *social supports*. On the other hand, it is useful to ascertain *any factors that might protect her against self-harm*, e.g. pets and the fact that despite a long history of depression Miss Y has never tried to harm herself.

Management options

Social

As stated above, Miss Y is socially isolated and regular follow-up (e.g. weekly or fortnightly) is important in addition to encouraging the development of social supports. She is finding work difficult, so a medical certificate should be offered for an agreed period of time (e.g 1 month), with the explanation that this can be extended as necessary. It is important to inform Miss Y that a diagnosis of depression will be recorded on her medical certificate.

Drug treatment

Drug treatment should be advised because Miss Y has a recurrent depressive illness at the more severe end of the spectrum. However, a number of issues need to be considered:

- Safety profile – It must be remembered that TCAs are cardiotoxic in overdose and if there is any concern about risk of overdose they should be given in small amounts (e.g. 1 or 2 days supply), supervised by a carer or avoided altogether. In the case of Miss Y, the risk of self-harm does not appear to be a major concern at present, but close monitoring of this is essential.
- Co-morbidity – Miss Y has complained of palpitations and TCAs are contraindicated in patients with arrhythmias. A thorough medical assessment should be carried out to exclude an arrhythmia (e.g. consider ECG, other cardiac investigations and possible referral to a cardiologist). Consider the possibility that the palpitations may be related to anxiety. If a cardiac problem is identified an alternative antidepressant should be considered (e.g. SSRI).
- Drug interactions – A pharmacokinetic/pharmacodynamic interaction between chlorpromazine and TCAs (both have cardiac effects) may be responsible for the palpitations and it would be wiser to avoid chlorpromazine. Another option would be to change the TCA to an SSRI or another antidepressant.
- Drug history – It is important to obtain a detailed antidepressant history, including what drugs have been tried in the past, the doses used, compliance and duration of treatment and any side-effects experienced with the different drugs. Miss Y has told you that she did not benefit from SSRIs in the past, but it may be that Miss Y didn't take these for an adequate period of time (6 weeks).
- Class of antidepressant and dose – From the history, Miss Y has been treated with both SSRIs and TCAs, although she claims that SSRIs did not help her depression. The current dose of amitriptyline is relatively low and clearly has failed to prevent a relapse. Provided her cardiac condition allows

continuing of the TCA therapy and the patient can tolerate potential side-effects, it is advisable to gradually increase the dose, aiming for an average of 150 mg a day.

- Side-effect profile of antidepressant – Any potential side-effects should be explained to the patient *before* starting treatment. Patient education about how to take antidepressants, how they work and potential side-effects that may be experienced will help improve compliance with treatment. This should include written information (e.g. a leaflet) when possible.

Psychological

The diagnosis of depression should be discussed with Miss Y and reassurance given that the illness is treatable.

Evidence of the benefit of psychological therapies (e.g. CBT, problem-solving therapy, counselling, IPT) is more dubious for patients with more severe depression, but they may be helpful once the patient starts to improve (usually because of antidepressants). Antidepressants should be regarded as the mainstay of treatment, but Miss Y should be offered psychological treatment as an adjunct to medication during her illness.

Follow-up

Consideration should be given to long-term treatment, and follow-up for this patient and consultation with the specialist services will be helpful.

Case 3

History

Mrs A is a 70-year-old lady who had a diagnosis of depression made 18 months ago and since that time she has been taking lofepramine (70 mg daily). There was no previous history of depression and Mrs A was fully independent at home.

Mrs A's daughter, who has just returned from a 2-week holiday and is concerned about her mother's mental state, calls you to do a home visit. Mrs A is refusing to get out of bed, her flat is in a mess and she is refusing to eat, claiming that her food is being poisoned. She is also saying that she wants to die and is thinking about taking all her tablets at once, but she isn't sure whether these would be enough to kill her.

There is no history of alcohol use. Her medical history includes non-insulin-dependent diabetes mellitus and chronic obstructive airway disease. Mrs A's aunt had a manic–depressive illness.

Discussion

Diagnosis

Mrs A has developed a depressive illness for the first time in old age. It is important to exclude an underlying physical cause for her symptoms (e.g. drugs, alcohol, carcinoma, infection, endocrine and metabolic disease, and neurological disease, e.g. Parkinson's disease and dementia). A thorough physical (including neurological) examination should be performed. Investigations should include routine blood (full blood count, erythrocyte sedimentation rate, urea and electrolytes and liver function tests) as well as vitamin B12 and serum/red cell folate and thyroid function tests and a CT brain scan. Mrs A appears to have psychotic symptoms in the form of paranoid delusions (she is convinced that her food is poisoned). These may be due to the depressive illness itself, another psychotic illness or an organic cause. A common cause of acute onset of delusions in the elderly is infection and the possibility of an acute confusional state should be excluded.

Triage

If the diagnosis is confirmed as psychotic depression, this is clearly severe, and Mrs A will need pharmacological treatment.

Risk assessment

Mrs A has multiple risk factors for self-harm: she is suicidal and has made a plan to overdose, she is not eating and she is psychotic. Mrs A needs to be admitted immediately to a psychiatric unit for observation and treatment. If she refuses voluntary hospital admission, consideration should be given to the use of the Mental Health Act.

Management options

Drug treatment

Mrs A will need treating in a psychiatric unit with antipsychotic and antidepressant medication. Electroconvulsive therapy may also be considered because this is particularly effective for the treatment of psychotic depression.

- Choice of antidepressant – Mrs A was taking lofepramine (a TCA). Lofepramine is a good choice of antidepressant for the elderly because it has fewer anticholinergic side-effects than other TCAs and it also has a good safety profile in overdose. In general, TCAs are *not* recommended for use in the elderly because of their tendency to cause anticholinergic side-effects and their potential for cardiotoxicity; however, sometimes their sedative effects are useful if given in low doses. SSRIs are a reasonable alternative to lofepramine for the elderly.
- Dose of antidepressant – Mrs A was only taking 70 mg lofepramine daily, which would be considered a subtherapeutic dose for a young, fit adult. However, the recommended dose of antidepressant is often lower for the

elderly, particularly if they are physically frail. In her case it appears that this dose was insufficient, as it failed to control her symptoms and allowed considerable worsening of her condition. The options are therefore either to increase the dose of lofepramine or change to an alternative antidepressant.

Social

Mrs A will need a strong support network once she is discharged from hospital. Her family supports will need investigating and she is likely to need help, at least initially, from social services (home help, meals on wheels may need consideration). Day-centre care may also be considered, along with follow-up from a community psychiatric nurse (CPN). An occupational therapist home assessment and multidisciplinary case conference should be considered prior to discharge.

Psychological

Community mental-health services should be involved, at least in the short term, following hospital discharge. They will provide regular follow-up and allow early identification of any problems. Mrs A is unlikely to require psychological therapy if she is followed up regularly by the CPN team, although the option should be discussed once her depressive symptoms have improved with medication. Psychological therapies have been shown to be as effective in the elderly as in younger patients,[60] although this is in the short term and for patients with mild to moderate depression.

An assessment of her cognitive state is essential once her depression is under control to exclude an underlying dementing illness.

References

1. Lepine JP, for the DEPRES Steering Committee. European perspective on depression. *Primary Care Psychiat* 1997; **3**(Suppl 1): S3–S6.

2. Freeling P, Rao BM, Paykel ES, Sireling LI, Burton RH. Unrecognised depression in general practice. *Br Med J* 1985; **290**: 1880–1883.

3. Rost K, Zhang M, Fortney J, Smith J, Coyne J, Smith-GR J. Persistently poor outcomes of undetected major depression in primary care. *Gen Hosp Psych* 1998; **20**: 12–20.

4. Ronalds C, Creed F, Stone K, Webb S, Tomenson B. The outcome of anxiety and depressive disorders in general practice. *Br J Psychiat* 1997; **171**: 427–433.

5. Simon GE, Goldberg D, Tiemens BG, Ustun TB. Outcomes of recognized and unrecognized depression in an international primary care study. *Gen Hosp Psychiat* 1999; **21**: 97–105.

6. Martucci M, Balestrieri M, Bisoffi G *et al*. Evaluating psychiatric morbidity in a general hospital: a two-phase epidemiological survey. *Psychol Med* 1999; **29**(4): 823–832.

7. Isaacsson G, Boethius G, Bergman U. Low level of an antidepressant prescription for people who later commit suicide: 15 years of experience from a population based drug database in Sweden. *Acta Psychiat Scand* 1992; **85**(6): 444–448.

8. Tylee A, Gastpar M, Lepine JP, Mendlewitz J. DEPRES II (Depression Research in European Society II): a patient survey of the symptoms, disability, and current management of depression in the community. DEPRES Steering Committee. *Int Clin Psychopharmacol* 1999; **14**(3): 139–151.

9. Murphy JM, Laird NM, Monson RR, Sobol AM, Leighton AH. A 40-year perspective on the prevalence of depression. The Stirling County Study. *Arch Gen Psychiat* 2000; **57**: 209–215.

10. Davidson JR, Meltzer-Brody SE. The underrecognition and undertreatment of depression: what is the breadth and depth of the problem? *J Clin Psychiat* 1999; **60**(7): 4–9; discussion 10–11.

11. Kind P, Sorensen J. The costs of depression. *Int Clin Psychopharmacol* 1993; **7**(3/4): 191–195.

12. Greenberg PE, Stiglin LE, Finkelstein SN *et al*. The economic burden of depression in 1990. *J Clin Psychiat* 1993; **54**: 405–418.

13. Eaton WW, Kramer M, Anthony JC *et al*. The incidence of specific DIS/DSM-III mental disorders: data from the NIMH Epidemiologic Catchment Area Program. *Acta Psychiat Scand* 1989; **79**: 163–178.

14. Kessler RC, McGonagle KA, Zhao S *et al*. Lifetime and 12-month prevalence of DSM-IIIR psychiatric disorders in the United States. Results from the National Comorbidity Survey. *Arch Gen Psychiat* 1994; **51**: 8–19.

15. Jenkins R, Bebbington B, Brugha TS, Farrell M, Lewis G, Meltzer H. British psychiatric morbidity survey. *Br J Psychiat* 1998; **173**: 4–7.

16. McLoone P, Crombie IK. Hospitalisation for deliberate self-poisoning in Scotland from 1981 to1993: trends in rates and types of drugs used. *Br J Psychiat* 1996; **169**: 81–85.

17. Angst J. How recurrent and predictable is depressive illness? In: Montgomery SA, Rouillon F, editors. *Long-term Treatment of Depression*. Chichester: John Wiley, 1992; pp. 1–13.

18. Angst J. Clinical course of affective disorders. In: Helgason T, Daly RJ, editors. *Depressive Illness: Prediction of Course and Outcome*. Berlin: Springer, 1988; pp. 1–48.

19. Kessing LV. "Recurrence in affective disorder, II: Effect of age and gender". *Br J Psychiat* 1998; **172**: 29–34.

20. Boulenger J-P, Lavalle Y-J. Mixed anxiety and depression: diagnostic issues. *J Clin Psychiat* 1993; **54**(Suppl 1): 3–8.

21. Duggan C, Sham P, Minne C, Lee A, Murray R. Family history as predictor of poor long-term outcome in depression. *Br J Psychiat* 1998; **173**: 527–530.

22. Andrew M, McGuffin P, Katz R. Genetic and non-genetic subtypes of major depressive disorder. *Br J Psychiat* 1998; **173**: 523–526.

23. Falconer DS. The inheritance of liability to certain diseases estimated from the incidence among relatives. *Ann Human Genet* 1965; **29**: 51–76.

24. Paykel ES, Myers JK, Dienelt MN, Klerman GL, Lindenthal JJ, Pepper MP. Life events and depression. A controlled study. *Arch Gen Psychiat* 1969; **21**: 753–760.

25. Birley JLT, Brown GW. Social precipitants of severe psychiatric disorders. *Psychiat Epidemiol* 1970; 321–325. London: Oxford University Press, for Nuffield Provincial Hospitals Trust.

26. Cooper B, Sylph J. Life events and the onset of neurotic illness: an investigation in general practice. *Psychol Med* 1973; **3**: 421–435.

27. Brown GW *et al*. Life events and psychiatric disorders. 1. Some methodological issues. *Psychol Med* 1973; **3**: 74–87.

28. Brown GW *et al*. Life events and psychiatric disorders. 2. Nature of causal link. *Psychol Med* 1973; **3**: 159–176.

29. Brown GW, Harris T. *Social Origins of Depression*. Tavistock: London, 1978.

30. Henderson S. The social network, support and neurosis. *Br J Psychiat* 1977; **131**: 185–191

31. Kawachi I, Berkman LF. Social ties and mental health. *J Urban Health* 2001; **78**(3): 458–467.

32. Wilkinson RG. Health, hierachy, and social anxiety. *Ann NY Acad Sci* 1999; **896**: 48–63.

33. Son SE, Kirchner JT. Depression in children and adolescents. *American Family Physician* 2000; **62**(10): 2297–2308, 2311–2312.

34. Weller EB, Weller RA. Depression in adolescents growing pains or true morbidity? *J Affective Disord* 2000; **61**(1): 9–13.

35. Lara ME, Klein DN. Psychosocial processes underlying the maintenance and persistence of depression: implications for understanding chronic depression. *Clin Psychol Rev* 1999; **19**(5): 553–570.

36. O'Hara MW. *Postpartum Depression: Causes and Consequences*. New York: Springer-Verlag, 1995.

37. Schildkraut JJ. The catecholamine hypothesis of affective disorders: review of supporting evidence. *Am J Psychiat* 1965; **122**: 509-522.

38. Coppen A. The biochemistry of affective disorders. *Br J Psychiat* 1967; **113**: 1237–1264.

39. Baxter LR, Schwartz JM, Phelps ME, Maziotta JC, Guze BH, Selin CE, Gerner RH, Sumida RM. Reduction of prefrontal cortex glucose metabolism common to three types of depression. *Arch Gen Psychiat* 1989; **46**: 243–250.

40. Nemeroff C. The corticotropin-releasing factor (CRF) hypothesis of depression: new findings and new directions. *Molec Psychiat* 1996; **1**: 336–342.

41. Lima MS, Moncrieff J. Drugs versus placebo for dysthymia (Cochrane review). *Cochrane Library* 1999, issue 4. Update Software: Oxford.

42. Kendrick T, Burns T *et al.* Provision of care to general practice patients with disabling long term mental illness. *BJGP* 1994; **44**: 301–305.

43. Goldberg D, Huxley P. *Common Mental Disorders; A Biosocial Model.* London: Tavistock/Routledge, 1992.

44. Hickie IB, Davenport TA, Scott EM, Hadzi-Pavlovic D, Naismith SL, Koschera A. Unmet need for recognition of common mental disorders in Australian General Practice. *Med J Aust* 2001; **175**(Suppl): S18–S24.

45. Grimshaw JM, Russell IT. Effect of clinical guidelines on medical practice: a systematic review of rigorous evaluations. *Lancet* 1993; **342**: 1317–1322.

46. Stevens L, Kinmonth AL, Peveler R, Thompson C. The Hampshire Depression Project: development and piloting of clinical practice guidelines and education about depression in primary health care. *Med Educat* 1997; **31**: 375–379.

47. Paykel ES, Hart D, Priest RG. Changes in public attitudes to depression during the Defeat Depression Campaign. *Br J Psychiat* 1998; **173**: 519–522.

48. Oxman T, Barrett T, Barrett J, Garter P. Symptomatology of late-life minor depression among primary care patients. *Psychosomatics* 1990; **31**: 174–180.

49. Mayou R. Depression and types of physical disorder and treatment. In: Robertson MM, Katona CLE, editors. *Depression and Physical Illness.* Chichester: John Wiley, 1997; pp. 21–38.

50. Weissman MM, Bland RC, Canino GJ *et al.* Cross-national epidemiology of major depression and bipolar disorder. *J Am Med Assoc* 1996; **276**: 293–299.

51. Gillam SJ, Jarman B, White P, Law R. Ethnic differences in consultation rates in urban general practice. *Br Med J* 1989; **299**: 953–957.

52. Kawanishi Y. Somatization of Asians: an artefact of Western medicalization? *Transcultural Psychiatr Res Rev* 1992; **29**: 5–36.

53. Simon GE, VonKorff M, Piccinelli M *et al.* An international study of the relation between somatic symptoms and depression. *New Engl J Med* 1999; **341**: 1329–1336.

54. Kirmayer LJ, Robbins JM, Dworkind M *et al.* Somatization and the recognition of depression and anxiety in primary care. *Am J Psychiat* 1993; **150**: 734–741.

55. Garcia-Campayo J, Lobo A, Perez-Echeverria MJ *et al*. Three forms of somatization presenting in primary care settings in Spain. *J Nerv Ment Dis* 1998; **186**: 554–560.

56. Hull S, Cornwell J, Harvey C, Eldridge S. Prescribing rates for psychotropic medication amongst east London general practices: low rates where Asian populations are greatest. *Family Practice* 2000; **18**(2): 167–172.

57. Cinnirella M, Loewenthal KM. Religious and ethnic group influences on beliefs about mental illness: a qualitative interview study. *Br J Med Psychol* 1999; **72**(4): 505–524.

58. Ustun TB, Goldberg D, Cooper J, Simon GE, Sartorius N. New classification for mental disorders with management guidelines for use in primary care. *BJGP* 1995; **45**: 211–215.

59. Dowrick C, Dunn G, Ayuso-Mateos J, Dalgard O, Page H, Lehtinen V, Casey P, Wilkinson C, Vazquez-Barquero J, Wilkinson G and the Outcomes of Depression International Network (ODIN) Group. Problem solving treatment and group psychoeducation for depression: multicentre randomised controlled trial. *Br Med J* 2000; **321**: 1450–1454.

60. Department of Health. Treatment choice in psychological therapies and counselling: evidence based clinical practice guidelines. www.doh.gov.uk/mentalhealth/treatmentguideline; Department of Health, 2001.

61. Rowland N, Bower P, Mellor-Clark J *et al*. Counselling for depression in primary care (Cochrane Review). The Cochrane Library, Issue 2. Oxford: Update Software, 2001.

62. Hunot V, Churchill R, Corney R, Knapp M, McGuire H, Tylee A, Wessely S. A systematic review of controlled trials of the effectiveness and cost-effectiveness of brief psychological treatments for depression. Cochrane Review (in progress).

63. Weissman MM, Markowitz JC. Interpersonal psychotherapy: current status. *Arch Gen Psychiat* 1994; **51**: 599–606.

64. Freedman N. Hoffenberg JD. Vorus N. Frosch A. The effectiveness of psychoanalytic psychotherapy: the role of treatment duration, frequency of sessions, and the therapeutic relationship. *J Am Psychoanalytic Assoc* 1999; **47**(3): 741–772.

65. Thase ME. Psychotherapy of refractory depressions. *Depression Anxiety* 1997; **5**: 190–201.

66. Priest RG *et al.* Lay people's attitudes to treatment of depression: results of opinion poll for Defeat Depression Campaign just before its launch. *Br Med J* 1996; **313**: 858–859.

67. Robinson LA, Berman JS, Neimeyer RA. Psychotherapy for the treatment of depression: a comprehensive review of controlled outcome research. *Psychol Bull* 1990; **100**: 30–49.

68. Elkin I. *The NIMH Treatment of Depression Collaborative Research Program: where we began and where we are*. In: Bergin AE, Garfield SL, editors. *Handbook of Psychotherapy and Behavior Change*, 4th edition. New York: Wiley, 1994.

69. Quitkin FM, Harrison W, Stewart JW *et al.* Response to phenelzine and imipramine in placebo nonresponders with atypical depression: a new application of the crossover design. *Arch Gen Psychiat* 1991; **48**: 319–323.

70. Goodheart RS, Dunne JW, Edis RH. Phenelzine associated peripheral neuropathy: clinical and electrophysiological findings. *Aust NZ J Med* 1991; **21**: 339–340.

71. Versiani M, Nardi AE, Mundim FD *et al.* Pharmacotherapy of social phobia: a controlled study with moclobemide and phenelzine. *Br J Psychiat* 1992; **161**: 353–360.

72. Shoaf SE, Linnoila M. Interaction of ethanol and smoking on the pharmacokinetics and pharmacodynamics of psychotropic medications. *Psychopharmacol Bull* 1991; **27**: 577–594.

73. DeVane LC. Principles of pharmacokinetics and pharmacodynamics. In: Schatzberg AF, Nemeroff CB, editors. *Psychopharmacology*. Washington, DC: American Psychiatric Press, 1998; pp. 155–169.

74. Glassman AH, Roose SP, Bigger JT Jr. The safety of tricyclic antidepressants in cardiac patients: risk-benefit reconsidered. *J Am Med Assoc* 1993; **269**: 2673–2675.

75. Riddle MA, Geller B, Ryan N. Another sudden death in a child treated with desipramine. *J Am Acad Child Adolesc Psychiat* 1993; **32**: 792–797.

76. Anderson IM, Tomenson BM. The efficacy of selective serotonin reuptake inhibitors in depression: a meta-analysis of studies against tricyclic antidepressants. *J Psychopharmacol* 1994; **8**: 238–249.

77. Dawkins K, Potter WZ. Gender differences in pharmacokinetics and pharmacodynamics of psychotropics: focus on women. *Psychopharmacol Bull* 1991; **27**(4): 417–426.

78. Montgomery SA, Henry J, McDonald G, Dinan T, Lader M, Hindmarch I. Selective serotonin re-uptake inhibitors: meta-analysis of discontinuation rates. *Int Clin Psychopharmacol* 1994; **9**: 47–53.

79. Boyer WF, Feigner JP. Safety and tolerability of selective serotonin re-uptake inhibitors. In: Feigner JP, Boyer WF, editors. *Selective Serotonin Re-uptake Inhibitors: Advances in Basic Research and Clinical Practice*. Chichester: John Wiley, 1996; pp. 291–314.

80. Ciraulo DA, Shader RI. Fluoxetine drug–drug interactions. I: Antidepressants and antipsychotics. *J Clin Psychopharmacol* 1990; **10**: 48–50.

81. Crewe HK, Lennard MS, Tucker GT *et al*. The effect of selective serotonin reuptake inhibitors on the cytochrome P450IID6 activity in human liver microsomes. *Br J Clin Pharmacol* 1992; **34**: 262–265.

82. Sternbach H. The Serotonin syndrome. *Am J Psych* 1991; **148**: 705–713.

83. Lejoyeux M, Ades J, Rouillon F. Serotonin syndrome: incidence, symptoms and treatment. *CNS Drugs* 1994; **2**(2): 132–143.

84. Byrne SE, Rothschild AJ. Loss of antidepressant efficacy during maintenance therapy: possible mechanisms and treatments. *J Clin Psychiat* 1998; **59**: 279–288.

85. Frank E, Prien RF, Jarrett RB *et al*. Conceptualization and rationale for consensus definitions of terms in major depressive disorder: remission, recovery, relapse and recurrence. *Arch Gen Psychiat* 1991; **48**: 851–855.

Appendix 1 – Treatment Guide for Commonly Used Antidepressants and Common Side-effects

	Usual daily dose	Starting and usual treatment dose in the frail elderly (see current BNF for further details)	Common side-effects	Relative cost
Tricyclics and related antidepressants				
Amitriptyline	150 mg od	25–75 mg	S, ↓BP, AC, W	L
Dothiepin	150 mg od	50–75 mg	S, ↓BP, AC, W	L
Imipramine	150 mg od	10–50 mg	↓BP, AC, S, W	L
Lofepramine	70 mg bd	70–105 mg	AC	L–M
SSRIs				
Citalopram (Cipramil)	20 mg od	10–30 mg	N	M
Fluoxetine (Prozac)	20 mg od	10 (alt. days)–20 mg	N	L–M
Fluvoxamine (Faverin)	100–200 mg od	100–200 mg	N, S	
Paroxetine (Seroxat)	20 mg od	10–20 mg	N, W	M
Sertraline (Lustral)	50–100 mg od	25–75 mg	N	M
Others				
Mirtazapine (Zispin)	30 mg od	15 mg	S, W	M
Moclobemide (Manerix)	150 mg bd	–	I	M
Nefazodone (Dutonin)	200 mg bd	100 mg bd	S	M
Reboxetine(Edronax)	(4 mg bd)	Avoid	I	M
Venlafaxine (Efexor)	37.5 mg bd	75 mg	↑BP, W	M–H

Key: AC = anticholinergic; BP = blood pressure; I = insomnia; N = nausea; S = sedation; W = weight gain; L = low; M = medium; H = high.

St John's wort

There is some evidence to suggest that St John's wort (*Hypericum perforatum*) may be effective for the short-term treatment of patients with mild to moderate depressive illness. However,

- Further studies are necessary before recommending the use of St John's wort as an antidepressant.
- St John's wort has pharmacological actions similar to antidepressant drugs and should not be used in combination with these, as there is danger of drug interactions!

Appendix 2 – Summary of Side-effects of Antidepressant Drugs

Antidepressant	Sedation	Weight	Sexual dysfunction	Seizure threshold	Heart rate	Blood pressure	Direct cardiac effects
TCAs	++ (varies with different TCAs)	↑	+	↓↓ (dose related, particularly maprotiline)	↑	Orthostatic hypotension ↑BP in toxicity	+
SSRIs	±	– or ↓ ↑ (less common)	++	↓		–	–
MAOIs	±	+ (phenelzine)	++	–	±	+	–
Reboxetine	–	–	±		±	±	–
Venlafaxine	–	–	+	↓	+	↑ (higher doses)	–
Trazodone	+	±	±	↓*	±	↓	–
Nefazodone	+	±	–	↓*	–	–	–
Mirtazapine	++	++	–	↓*	–	– ↓	–

↓* - low incidence.

Appendix 3 – Useful Addresses and Websites

For the primary care physician

Societies, journals and congresses

World Psychiatric Association
Address: International Center for Mental Health, Mount Sinai School of Medicine, of New York University - Fifth Avenue & 100th Street, Box 1093 New York, NY 10029-6574 USA
Tel.: +1 718 334 5094, +1 718 334 3459
Fax: +1 718 334 5096
E-mail: wpa@dti.net
Website: www.wpanet.org
Congress: World Congress of Psychiatry (annual)

The American Psychiatric Association
Address: 400 K Street N.W., Washington, DC 20005, USA
Tel.: +1 888 357 7924
Fax: +1 202 682 6850
E-mail: apa@psych.org
Website: www.psych.org

The National Institute of Mental Health
Addresses: NIMH Public Inquiries, 6001 Executive Boulevard, Rm. 8184, MSC 9663, Bethesda, MD 20892-9663 USA
Tel.: +1 301 443-4513
Fax: +1 301 443-4279
E-mail: nimhinfo@nih.gov
Website: www.nimh.nih.gov

National Alliance for Research on Schizophrenia and Depression (NARSAD)
60 Cutter Mill Road, Suite 404, Great Neck, NY 11021 USA
Tel.: +1 516 829-0091
Fax: +1 516 487-6930
Infoline: +1 800 829 8289
Research Grants Program: +1 516 829-5576
E-mail: info@narsad.org
Website: www.mhsource.com/narsad/

National Depressive and Manic-Depressive Association (DMDA)
Address: 730 N. Franklin Street, Suite 501, Chicago, Illinois 60610-7204 USA
Tel: +1 312 642 0049
Fax: +1 312 642-7243
Toll Free: 800 826 3632

National Mental Health Association
Address: 1021 Prince Street, Alexandria, Virginia 22314-2971, USA
Tel.: +1 703 684-7722,
Toll Free: 800 969-NMHA (6642)
TTY: 800 433-5959
Fax: +1 703 684-5968

Royal College of Pyschiatrists
17 Belgrave Square, London SW1X 8PG, UK
Tel: +44 (0) 20 7235 2351
Fax: +44 (0) 20 7245 1231
E-mail: webmaster@rcpsych.ac.uk
Website: www.rcpsych.ac.uk
Journal: The British Journal of Psychiatry
Congress: The Royal College of Psychiatrists Annual Meeting (annual)

The Canadian Psychiatric Association
260-441 MacLaren Street, Ottawa, Ontario, K2P-2H3, Canada
Tel.: +1 613 234 2815
Fax: +1 613 234 9857
E-mail: cpa@cpa-apc.org
Website: www.cpa-apc.org
Journal: The Canadian Journal of Psychiatry (cjp@cpa-apc.org)
Congress: Annual Meeting (agm@cpa-apc.org)

For the Patient

National Foundation For Depressive Illness, Inc.
P.O. Box 2257, New York, NY 10116
Tel: +1 800 239 1265
Website: www.depression.org

Manic Depression Fellowship
Address: MDF National Office, Castle Works, 21 St. George's Road, London SE1 6ES UK
Tel.: +44 (0) 20 7793 2600
Fax: +44 (0) 20 7793 2639.
E-mail: mdf@mdf.org.uk
Website: www.mdf.org.uk

MDF (Wales)
Address: 1 Palmyra Place, Newport, Gwent NP20 4EJ
Tel.: +44 (0) 1633 244244
Fax: +44 (0) 1633 244111.
E-mail: mdfwales@btconnect.com
Website: www.manicdepressionwales.org.uk

MDF (Scotland)
Address: 7 Woodside Crescent, Glasgow G3 7UL
Tel.: +44 (0) 141 400 1867
Fax: +44 (0) 141 331 0366

Depression Alliance
Address: 35 Westminster Bridge Road, London SE1 7JB
Tel.: +44 (0) 207 633 0557
Fax: +44 (0) 207 633 0559
Website: www.depressionalliance.org

Fellowship of Depressives Anonymous
Address: FDA c/o Self Help Nottingham, Ormiston House, 32-36 Pelham, Street, Nottingham, NG1 2EG, UK
Tel.: +44 (0) 1702 433838
Fax : +44 (0) 1702 433843
Website: ww.edinburgh.gov.uk/HEBS/UK_Health_Advice_Groups_FELLOWSHIP_OF_DEPRESSIVES_ANONYMOUS_FDAhtml

MIND – National Association for Mental Health
Address: Branta House, 15–19 Broadway, Stratford, London E15 4BQ, UK
Tel.: +44 (0) 20 8519 2122 MindinfoLine 08457 660 163
Website: www.mind.org.uk

Scottish Association for Mental Health
Address: Cumbrae House, 15 Carlton Court, Glasgow G5 9JP
Tel.: +44 (0) 141 568 7000
Fax: +44 (0) 141 568 7001
Email: enquire@samh.org.uk
Website: www.samh.org.uk

The Samaritans
Address: The Upper Mill, Kingston Road, Ewell, Surrey KT17 2AF
Tel.: Enquiries 020 8394 8300
Helpline: 08457 90 90 90 (UK), +1 850 60 90 90 (RoI)
Fax: 020 8394 8301
Website: www.samaritans.org.uk

Association for Postnatal Illness
Address: 145 Dawes Road, Fulham, London, UK, SW6 7EB Tel.: 020 7386 0868
Tel.: +44 (0) 20 7386 0868 (UK)
Fax: +44 (0) 20 7386 8885
Website: www.apni.org
E-mail: info@apni.org

British Association for Counselling and Psychotherapy (BACP)
Address: 1 Regent Place, Rugby, Warks CV21 2PJ
Tel.: +44 (0) 870 443 5252
Fax: +44 (0) 870 443 5160
Minicom: +44 (0) 870 443 5162
E-mail: bac@bac.co.uk
Website: www.bacp.co.uk

African-Caribbean Mental Health Association
Address: 35–37 Electric Avenue, Brixton, London SW9 8JP
Tel.: +44 (0) 20 7737 3603

Index

***Note**: As depression is the subject of the book, all index entries refer to depression unless otherwise indicated. Page numbers followed by 'f' indicate figures; page numbers followed by 't' indicate tables. This index is in letter-by-letter order, whereby spaces and hyphens in main entries are excluded by the alphabetization process*

Abbreviations:
MAOIs = monoamine oxidase inhibitors
SSRIs = selective serotonin re-uptake inhibitors
TCAs = tricyclic antidepressants